CURE

ACHES AND PAINS THROUGH OSTEOPATHY

Dr. Krishna M. Modi
M.B.B.S., M.L. COM. (LONDON).
M.R.O. (ENGLAND)

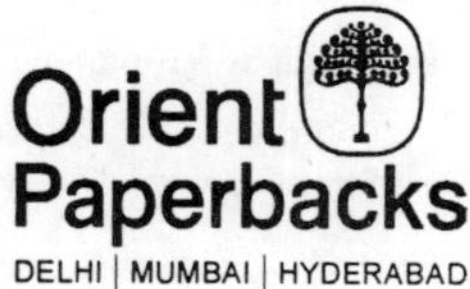

DELHI | MUMBAI | HYDERABAD

ISBN : 978-81-222-0211-3

Cure Aches and Pains Through Osteopathy

Subject: Health & Fitness / Massage & Reflexotherapy

1st Published 1997
10th Printing 2017

Published by
Orient Paperbacks
(A division of Vision Books Pvt. Ltd.)
5A/8 Ansari Road, New Delhi-110 002
www.orientpaperbacks.com

Cover Design by Vision Studio

Printed at
Yash Printographics, Noida

Printed on Chlorine-free eco-friendly paper.

Acknowledgements

I take this opportunity to express my gratitude to those who have assisted me with this book. First of all, I thank my teacher Dr S.M. Tuli, Professor and Head of the Department of Orthopaedics, Institute of Medical Sciences, Varanasi, who guided and encouraged me. Though we often differed in our thinking, we were imbued with the common objective of relieving suffering.

I am thankful to George W. Northup, Editor, Journal of the American Osteopathic Association, for his advice.

I thank my friend Dr Claude S. Dutton, LRCP, MRCS, DA, LLCO, who made his collection of worldwide publications on osteopathy available to me. My gratitude to Dr Thomas G. Dummer, DO, a believer in the use of *specific* and *less force* during manipulation for better results, and Dr Jamshed P. Randeria, LLCO, for acquainting me with the orthopaedic developments in UK.

A special thank you to my father Vithal Das Modi without whose encouragement and guidance this work would not have been possible.

My gratitude to my wife Usha whose endurance, untiring co-operation and support helped to make this book a reality.

A big thank you to my patients who put their firm belief in treatment by manipulation. And last, but not the least, I extend my appreciation to all those who by word and deed are helping osteopathy to get a firmer footing in this country.

Preface

After completing my MBBS, I joined the Central Institute of Orthopaedics, Safdarjung Hospital, New Delhi, as a house surgeon. This is a leading orthopaedic centre in India. To me, orthopaedics seemed a rewarding branch of medicine to specialise in. A person gets involved in a severe accident, fractures a bone, and comes to the orthopaedic department. The doctor examines him and confirms that he has suffered a fracture. The X-ray taken also confirms the diagnosis. Bones are manipulated under anaesthesia, placed in position, and the plaster is applied. Once again an X-ray is taken to confirm that the bones are in place. After six weeks the plaster is removed, and the broken bones are one again. The patient expresses his gratitude. The doctor is happy because his hands have been able to help somebody. His job satisfaction is complete.

This is the 'emergency' face of orthopaedics. Let us now examine the less dramatic side. Here we deal with patients suffering from backache, sciatica, lumbago, cervical spondylosis and other pains of the spine and the joints. The story is not the same. The patient comes with acute and chronic pains. All possible investigations are carried out. In most cases a diagnosis is made, but the treatment remains unsatisfactory. In spite of the genuine efforts of the doctor, the recovery often remains incomplete. The patient keeps coming week after week, month

Cure Aches and Pains through Osteopathy

osteopathy *n.* a system of healing based on the theory that many diseases are associated with disorders of the musculoskeletal system. Diagnosis and treatment of these disorders involve palpation, manipulation, and massage.

Oxford Concise Medical Dictionary, 3rd ed.

os-te-op-a-thy. a system of therapy based on the theory that the body is capable of making its own remedies against disease and other toxic conditions . . . emphasizes the importance of normal body mechanics and manipulative methods of detecting and correcting faulty structure.

Dorland's Pocket Medical Dictionary, 25th ed.

Increasingly, and across the globe, doctors, orthopaedic surgeons, physical medicine consultants and hospitals are acknowledging the effectiveness of osteopathy. Using body massage and bone manipulation techniques this therapy is being used to treat a variety of pains and aches, from backaches, including lumbago and sciatica, knee and elbow pain, and frozen shoulder to cervical spondylosis, headaches and migraine.

Using examples, illustrations and case histories, the book prescribes simple exercises which can be done at home to relieve aches, pains and a number of other discomforts associated with joint problems, bone degeneration and old age. It suggests when, where and the kind of manipulation required to treat a problem by minimising the use of drugs and avoiding surgical options.

This lucid and easy-to-follow book by India's foremost osteopath is invaluable for preventing, treating and curing all kinds of pains, aches and other related health problems.

The Author

Dr Krishna Murari Modi is a leading osteopath and, perhaps, the first one to qualify from India. He was a practising orthopaedist within the tradition of allopathy till he found himself dissatisfied with the inadequacy of this method in treating various types of aches and pains. He delved deeper and discovered that osteopathy, a therapy which could give tremendous relief to the sufferer, remained untapped.

Widely travelled through the US — the birthplace of osteopathy, European and Scandinavian countries, the erstwhile USSR and the Middle East, the author has gained firsthand knowledge of the latest advances in manipulative therapy. He has also written extensively on the subject.

He now runs a 100-bed hospital of alternative medicine — Dr Modi's Karjat Health Resort at Karjat, Village Wanjale, Dist. Raigarh, Maharashtra. He plans to open a training centre for osteopathy and natural medicine shortly.

after month, and feels frustrated at the doctor's inability to help despite all available knowledge. What is missing? I started looking for new methods to help. I read about the manipulation of the spine and different joints. But I wondered why we did not practise this method.

This was the time when newspapers were filled with the news of osteopath Stephen Ward, who was involved in the sensational Christine Keeler case along with several bigwigs in Britain including Profumo, a British cabinet minister. Profumo had to resign because of his involvement in the case. The news ended in the tragic suicide of Mr Ward. This was the year 1965. As I read the name of the osteopath again and again, I wanted to know what osteopathy was. I learned that osteopaths relieve their patients of aches and pain by manipulation.

I remember a story my grandmother used to tell us.

> Once upon a time there lived a king. He had a severe backache. He would turn, toss and roll in bed because of the severity of the pain. He would not allow anybody to touch him. This went on for a long time in spite of the best ministrations of the royal physician. The physician was worried. Several physicians from all parts of the country were summoned and an award was declared for the one who would cure him. All efforts were in vain. Ultimately a physician arrived from far off. He ordered the royal horse to be kept without food or water for four days. The horse was then brought to the king who, after some persuasion, was asked to mount it. The thirsty animal noticed water in a ditch and galloped towards it. As he bent his head to drink, the king gripped hard to save himself from falling. In the process the king's back clicked — and he was cured.

I was keen to learn manipulation. To my surprise, it was not a routine practice in our department. Manipulation under general anaesthesia was a rare occurrence. I decided to go abroad to study more about it.

In London, I sought out orthopaedic surgeons, consultants in physical medicine and osteopaths. I watched them manipulate their patients and became convinced about the efficacy of osteopathic manoeuvres.

I joined the London College of Osteopathy. The secretary of the college, Mr A. F. Lockwood, admitted that osteopathy ought to be grateful to the ill-fated Dr Ward — he had made osteopathy known all over the world.

Two interesting historical cases relating to manipulation may be mentioned.

Doctor Corvisort, the physician-in-chief of Napoleon and his wife, used to visit the royal couple twice a week. The Emperor enjoyed good health, so the physician's services were required only rarely. But one day Napoleon began suffering from violent lumbago. The doctor, who was summoned, asked Napoleon to disrobe and lie across a table. He then administered a sound and well-aimed slap on his hips. The stunned Emperor turned in fury but during this movement the painful contracture of his lumbar muscles mercifully disappeared. The insolence of the celebrated physician was pardoned. This was the first example of successful manipulation recorded in history. The difficulty of finding the exact point of application of force in this manoeuvre makes us avoid it in practice. We use other manoeuvres which are not so spectacular but have an equal measure of success.

Hitler suffered from severe pain which could be relieved only by osteopathic treatment. During the 2nd World War, an osteopath was always at his side during front-line operations.

Why has manipulation been so little appreciated? This book is a humble effort towards acquainting people with the art and science of manipulation. My hope is that eventually we will have an osteopathic department in the medical colleges in our country.

Jolly-Maker Apartments No. 3,
Flat 14, 1st Floor,
Cuffe Parade, Bombay 400 005.

DR KRISHNA M. MODI

Contents

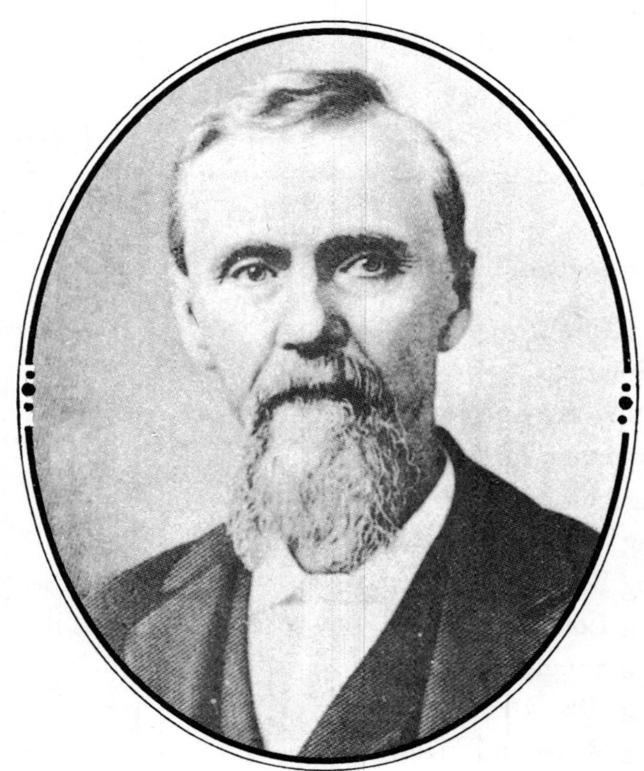

Dr Andrew Tailer Still

1
Growth of Osteopathy

Dr Andrew Tailer Still, the founder of osteopathy, was a man endowed with imagination, rare vision and perseverance.

He was born on August 6, 1828, to a simple, hardy German farmer who was a physician by training and a missionary by choice. His mother, Martha, was Scottish. Andrew was born in a remote village in Virginia, USA. He was sturdy and strong and lived close to nature. He was fond of watching different animals. He would catch hares and squirrels and dissect them to find out the type of organs they had.

Andrew's parents wanted him to become a Methodist minister. He wanted to be a physician, probably inspired by the visits he made with his father, assisting him on call of duty.

He describes an incident in his autobiography. He was ten years old when he got a severe headache. He was in agony. He took a rope and made a swing between two trees, about 6-8 inches above the ground, put a small pillow over it, placed his neck on it, and lay flat on the ground with his head hanging over the swing. He was reasonably comfortable that way. He went to sleep and got up twenty minutes later minus the headache. He knew nothing about the anatomy of the neck and he never imagined that this simple action with the swing could have stopped the headache. He used the same method till he was twenty years old. At this juncture he reasoned out his initial discovery: 'I could see that I had suspended the action of the great occipital nerves, and could give harmony to the flow of the arterial blood to and through the veins, and ease effect.'

Still joined the College of Physicians. When his wife Mary Vaugh died in 1859, he remarried and moved to an Indian settlement in Eastern Kansas. Later he joined the Army Medical Corps as a surgeon. At the end of the war, in October 1864, he was discharged from military service with the rank of Major. He resumed private practice. Medical science, at the time, was not very advanced and doctors made widespread use of mercurial preparations, irritants and alcohol. In 1875, a writer in a British medical journal advised diabetics to take mineral acids, bark and opium preparations. In the same issue Dr Conrad said that venereal diseases had some power to modify the eruptions of smallpox. Skin cancer was treated with arsenical paste, enuresis with Strychnine. In the light of modern medicine this was a foolish and dangerous trend.

At this juncture Still was hit by a great tragedy. Three of his sons died of spinal meningitis. He watched helplessly while his beloved children were snatched away by the cruel hands of Fate. This was the turning point in his life. His suspicion about the inadequacy of medical science was confirmed. He says in his autobiography: 'It was when I stood gazing at three members of my family all dead from spinal meningitis that I asked myself a serious question. In sickness had God left man stranded in a world of guessing? To guess what the matter was? To guess what to give and guess what the result would be? I decided then that God was not a guessing God but a God of truth. All his works, spiritual or material, were harmonious. So wise a God had certainly provided remedies for all illnesses.'

Still's own experience of curing his severe headache and his great personal tragedy drove him relentlessly towards a deeper study of Man. His anguish led him to the conviction that something must be found to enable the body to heal itself in accordance with the law of nature. He chose Baker University to present his new idea. His father and brothers had donated

480 acres of land to the university. When he approached the authorities with his new idea he was looked upon with raised eyebrows and his request to present his paper was turned down. In spite of the generosity of his family, his reputation as a good doctor, his career in the army and as a legislator, the university doors were closed to him.

His theory that the body possesses the power for self-healing and self-maintenance was not acceptable. Doctors continued to give patients opium and whisky, which was like adding poison to the body already loaded with toxins. Sir William Oster, a noted physician, said, 'He who takes medicine must get well twice, once from the disease he has and once from the medicines he has taken.'

Even this blow was not enough to make him deviate from his chosen path. He returned to Missouri and with greater determination went on developing his own theory. He maintained that the body was a complete unit and it was not possible for one part of the unit to be sick without affecting other parts. He believed in treating the body as a whole. He believed that the body's self-mechanism should be recognised and normalised, and this would do the rest of the job of prevention and treatment.

To understand disease we must know what health is and any deviation from it should be recognised. The muscular-skeletal system (constituting muscles, bones, ligaments and fascia) forms sixty per cent of the body mass. Unfortunately this part is most neglected. Any alteration or disorder in this system ought to affect the other systems of the body. The effect is mainly due to the nerve irritation which causes a muscle spasm, hence resulting in a change in blood supply and the flow of lymph.

Dr Still was hopeful and enthusiastic about his theories in spite of the criticism against him. In those days, to study human bones was a sin. Yet he went ahead and exhumed bodies from the shallow graves. He collected human bones and studied them in secrecy. The intricate mechanism of the human body fascinated and surprised him. He was curious about the sacro-iliac joint described in textbooks as a *joint which does not move.* He proved that the books were wrong. (Only recently have medical authorities arrived at the conclusion that the sacro-iliac joint has movement.) Then he examined the spine which is a great combination of flexibility and strength. Intricate bones preserve and protect the spinal chord and its branches. The nerves passing through the joints reach the muscles, joints and different organs. The spine has a disc between each joint which acts as a shock absorber.

Dr Still began to wonder why so many bones were so intricately interwoven, performing such delicate movements, and supporting the structure of the body. Would a change in the mechanism affect the body? If it was true that the change did affect the body, then he had found the cause.

He said, 'A thousand experiments were made with bones until I became quite familiar with the bony structure. I spent much time in the study of anatomy, physiology, chemistry and mineralogy. During the winters of 1878 and 1879 I was called to my old home in Kansas to treat a member of the family, whom I had doctored for ten years prior to my moving to Missouri. I treated partially by drugs, as was done in those days, but also gave osteopathic treatment and the patient got well.'

This was the start of the experiments on men. Dr Still started his new practice in Kirksville, Missouri, a small mid-west town. His critics did not give him any importance; instead, they looked upon him as a poor idealist doctor or an insane man.

This was also the time of great strides in medical science, when Lister was working on the theory of antisepsis, Pasteur on germ theory, and Virchow on physiology. The discovery of diphtheria antitoxins and the X-ray, however, came into use only years later.

Dr Still's theories stood the test of time. He experimented by fitting a stout bench-like table covered with leather in his office. It was long enough for a person to lie on, but not wide enough. The patients who came to him were placed on the table. After being physically examined, parts of their bodies were bent in different directions. Sensitive fingers would run over their spines; his hands would pause at tender areas; there would be quick movements and the pain was gone. They could not understand why a doctor would only push and pull to treat instead of administering a pill or a bottle of medicine. The relief experienced, however, began attracting a horde of patients. The news spread fast.

What part do nerves play in the symptom of a disease? Using bones as a leverage, how can one influence them? What role do arteries and veins play in the cure of a disease?

Dr Still concluded that blood supply could be normalised a great deal by manipulative manoeuvres which relaxed the muscles and thus affected the free flow of blood. He declared, 'The rule of the artery is supreme.' He was sure that the free flow of blood played a great role in overcoming disease.

Dr Still's fame spread gradually. At no time, however, did he think his discovery to be complete. With the co-operation of his sons and doctors who were attracted towards his science, he founded a new branch of medical treatment which came to be known as Osteopathic Medicine.

Dr Still planned to open a college of osteopathy. Assistance came in an astonishing way. Dr William Smith of Edinburgh, Scotland, was so impressed by Dr Still that he offered to stay and teach anatomy in exchange for lessons in manipulative movements. The college at Kirksville, Missouri, opened in November 1892, and was given legal recognition.

From the beginning, the main aim of the college was to improve medical practice. It was not a 'non-medical school.' Later it grew in stature and included all the arts and sciences of medical practice.

Kirksville became a centre of feverish activity. Patients flocked from far and near in big numbers; a few stayed on after getting cured to continue their studies. The college grew far beyond the hopes and imagination of Dr Still. New colleges were opened. Osteopathy was growing fast in USA and

UK. Dr Still passed his last few years sitting in the porch of his house on a hill overlooking the little town of Kirksville, where he could see the college building and hospital. A great experimenter, teacher and philosopher, he died on November 12, 1917. By then, more than 5,000 osteopathic physicians were practising in USA and other countries.

Still expounded that Man, a remarkable creation of God, was a self-sufficient, self-maintaining machine. The machine could run smoothly and look after itself. Osteopathy recognised this great self-healing and self-maintaining power of the man-machine.

It is not surprising that his theories evoked controversy. He was a complex man and his writings were difficult to understand. He could demonstrate and do things on his own, but could not put his ideas into writing in an organised form. His lectures used to be followed by demonstrations of his treatment on patients, without explaining much about what he could find and how he could put it right. A lot has been done since his time. Now there is a slow but definite recognition of Still's theories. He says in his *Philosophy of Osteopathy* that his great desire was to give a head start to a philosophy that could be a guide for the future. 'Great development in osteopathy today is the true emergence of his said philosophy.'

After Dr Still, osteopathy has produced many giants. They have contributed to its refinement and development. Today with many osteopathic hospitals, colleges and activities of different osteopathic associations in different countries, this branch of medicine is taking giant strides. Manipulative therapy, as medical science prefers to call it today, is becoming popular with medical men. Many doctors who suffer from pain themselves and ultimately get cured by manipulative therapy, try to learn a few techniques and apply them on their patients with astonishing results.

Manipulative treatment is part of the therapy as mentioned in orthopaedic textbooks. Osteopathy and chiropractic (where the same aim is achieved by using a slightly different technique) manipulation have come to be accepted as effective techniques of manipulative treatment. The truth, however, is that not everybody can be efficient and proficient in these techniques. A long time needs to be spent on self-training. Also there is the difficulty of finding an appropriate teacher. Techniques cannot be learnt by just studying books. Manipulation should be treated on par with other medical procedures. Who can deny the fact that even surgery saw black days beginning with the hands of barbers before the invention of anaesthesia!

Currently osteopathy is practised the most in the United States, its birth place. In UK, the profession had a relatively slower development. A few osteopaths from American colleges have settled in Australia. The Scandinavian countries are fast heading towards providing manipulative care to the public. There are quite a few osteopaths in France.

It was Dr J. B. Mannel (1877-1957) who first introduced gentle vertebral manipulation without anaesthesia within the domain of traditional medicine.

Recently the World Association of Natural Medicine came into existence. It includes osteopathy, chiropractic, acupuncture, hydrotherapy, naturopathy, yoga, hypnotism, meditation, physiotherapy and homoeopathy. Its head office is in Switzerland and a world conference is held there every year.

2
The Spine

It is very important to know the structure and functions of the spine before we begin to understand the cause of pain and what actually happens during manipulation. We must be familiar with the preventive methods and precautions we should take after the pain has gone so that we may not suffer from it again.

Understanding and becoming familiar with the anatomy or the structure of the human body is imperative to understand pathology or the disease process. Then only can we think of a remedy or treatment. Let us examine what our aim in manipulation is, and how these measures help to keep us healthy. Somebody has compared the human spine to a sitar and an osteopath to the maestro who plays the sitar. To learn the sitar, to master it, to produce new *ragas,* calls for a deep understanding and years of devoted practice. Appreciating the light and almost imperceptible touch and, at other times, the deep pressure applied on the strings, is what differentiates a maestro from an ordinary player. So it is with the skill of an osteopath. To manipulate the spine requires an equal amount of devotion and understanding added to years of an uninterrupted practice. The osteopath becomes a master of his job only after a devoted practice of at least five years after his graduation, during which he learns the basic knowledge only. It is also true that he never stops learning.

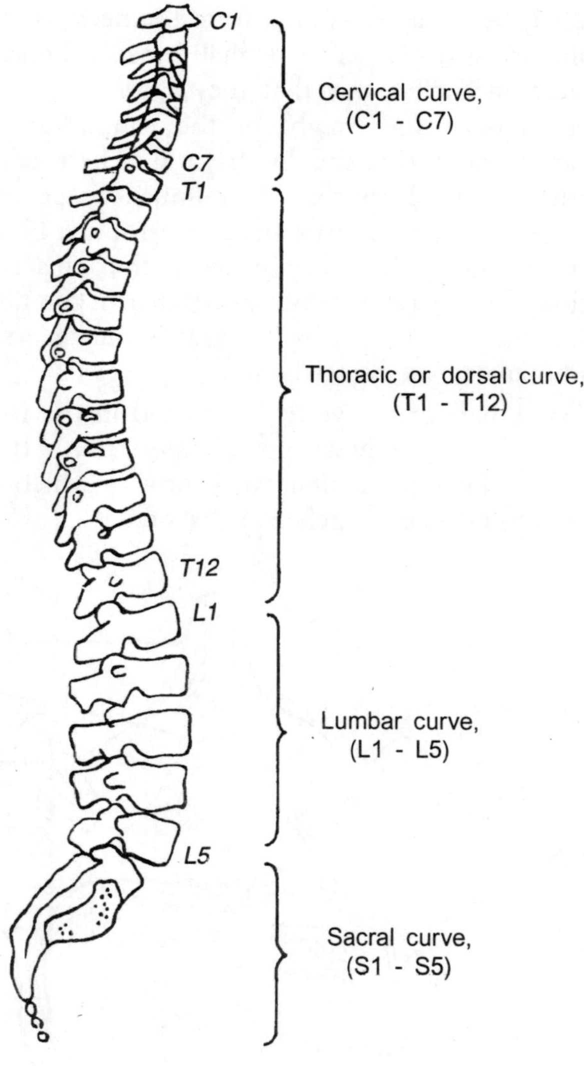

Fig. 1. The spine with its natural curves.

Man is a vertebrate. This means that he has a backbone called the spine, extending from the neck to the tail bone. The spine consists of a series of small irregular bones called vertebrae placed in such a way that they carry on different movements and support the weight of the trunk, thus making weight bearing easier for the lower limbs. These small bones called vertebrae are thirty-three in number. There are 7 vertebrae in the neck which comprise the cervical spine, 12 in the upper back comprising the dorsal spine, 5 in the loins called the lumbar spine. Five sacral bones fuse together in the tail bone region to form the sacrum, and below that is the coccyx formed by four rudimentary coccygeal bones.

The part of the vertebra situated in the front mainly helps to support the body weight. The posterior part called the neural arch, encloses the neural canal through which passes the spinal chord. The neural arch consists of:

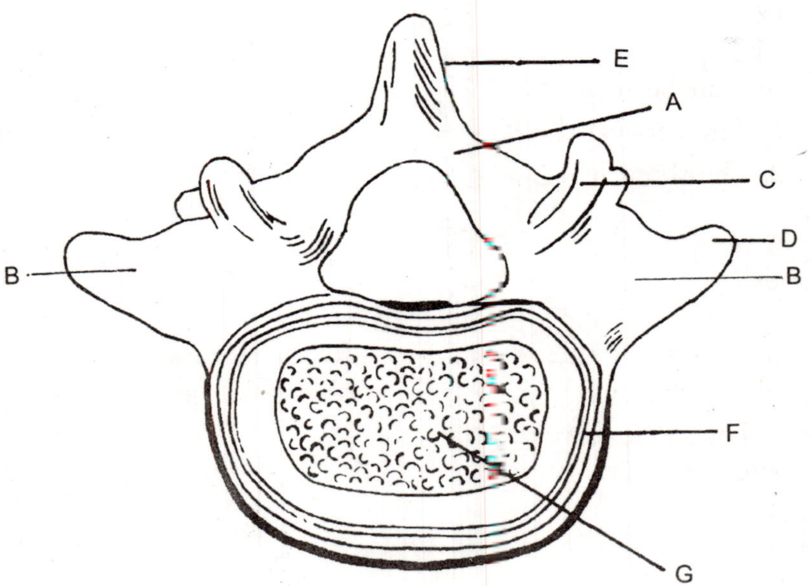

Fig. 2. A human vertebra. A. *Lamina;* B. *Spinous process;* C. *Articular facet;* D. *Transverse process;* E. *Pedicle;* F. *Annulus fibrosus;* G. *Nucleus pulposus.*

1. The pedicle or foot of the vertebra
2. A pair of transverse process or projections
3. Superior articular process or surfaces
4. Inferior articular process or surfaces
5. Spinous process
6. Laminae or lining covering the body of the vertebrae

The cervical spine has three peculiarities:

First, the transverse process of the cervical vertebrae is perforated by an opening through which pass the vertebral artery and the vein which supplies blood to the brain.

Second, the first cervical vertebra named Atlas supports the globe of the head and has no body.

Third, the second cervical vertebra called Axis provides the pivot upon which the atlas, the first vertebra, and the skull rotate.

Curves of the Spine

The spine is not straight. If it is viewed from a side, four curves can be seen (Fig. 1):

1. The cervical curve which is convex forward.

2. The thoracic curve which is concave forward. The upper part may have a slight lateral curvature directed towards the right side in a right-handed person and the left side in a left-handed person.

3. The lumbar curve is convex forward. It is more pronounced in females than males. It extends from the lower thoracic vertebra to the lumbo-sacral angle. It is larger than the upper two.

4. The pelvic curve extends from the lumbo-sacral joint to the apex of the coccyx. Its concavity faces downwards and forwards.

The vertebrae are held together and perform their functions of protection, movement and support.

The spine with the help of its inter-vertebral joints tries to perform the functions of movement and support in the best possible way.

Intervertebral Joints

Intervertebral joints are the joints between two adjacent vertebrae. They comprise the anterior joint-containing discs, the posterior joints constituted by facet or surface joints, a connecting ligament system, muscles, intervertebral foramen, and nerves.

Intervertebral Discs

The discs are interposed between the adjacent surfaces of the bodies of the vertebrae and form the chief bond of connection between them. Their shapes correspond with those of the bodies of the vertebrae between which they are lodged. Their thickness varies in different regions of the column and in different parts of the same disc. They are thicker in front in the cervical and lumbar region, thus constituting the anterior convexity of these curves. They are uniform in size in the thoracic region, and the anterior concavity of this column is due to the shape of the vertebral bodies, which are thinnest in the upper thoracic area and thickest in the lumbar region.

The disc absorbs the pressure transmitted to it by the central core, and, at the same time, keeps the vertebrae together. It buffers the action of compression upon bones. It is the chief shock absorber of the body. It constitutes one-fourth (quarter) of the entire length of the spine. The shock absorption is based more on the hydraulic system, also akin to the elastic properties of rubber.

The disc consists of 3 parts: the end plate, the peripheral portion called the annulus fibrosus, and the central portion called the nucleus pulposus.

The End Plate. This consists of a narrow zone of hyaline cartilage covering each surface of the vertebral body. The end plate, along with the annulus, is perforated by thousands of small holes through which the tissue fluid diffuses. The fluid diffuses both into and out of the disc.

The Annulus Fibrosus. The annulus fibrosus comprises the narrow outer zone of collagenous fibres and a wider inner zone of fibro-cartilage. It is attached to the end plates. Fibres of this layer run obliquely, thus giving great strength to the rotational movements. The annulus fibrosus surrounds the nucleus pulposus in the form of a number of layers which can be compared to the layers of an onion. Around its periphery the annulus inserts itself on the vertebral body. The marginal fibres are particularly tough. The weakest point is located at the posterior near the intervertebral foramen.

The disc is nourished by synovial fluid and if a piece flakes off, it remains alive inside the joint cavity. The cartilage has no nerve or blood supply. It is nourished by the bone of the body of the vertebrae. It is therefore slow to react to a trauma, and also slow and often incapable of complete repair. That is why there is no immediate pain if the cartilage is damaged. The pain is felt only when adjacent sensitive structures are also affected.

Following the trauma to any tissue, there is swelling owing to the liberation of histamine and other substances. The cartilage swells after the forced activity, but due to the lack of nerve supply, it does not cause pain, and due to the absence of blood supply, it swells up slowly. Two or more days following the injury may pass before the cartilage swells up. However, ligaments, if injured, swell up in 2-3 hours. The swelling may stretch to adjacent ligaments or the periosteum (outer layer of a bone), causing pain, or the swelling may block the full range of movements. Adequate rest required for the repair of the joint is usually not given to it. Repair is therefore often incomplete and consequently, degenerative changes in the annulus are induced much earlier than desired. All the damage to the annulus is permanent: a union and regeneration never take place here.

A disc has the quality of a sponge and is able to absorb fluid as well as diffuse its own fluid content. This is why the consistency of the disc keeps on changing. This can be demonstrated by measuring the height of a person at the end of the day and early in the morning when he gets up. The height of the person increases by ¼ to ¾ of an inch after a night's sleep. This height difference is not due to the straightening of the curves of the spine but due to an increase in the thickness of the discs.

The Nucleus Pulposus. This is a soft, gelatinous, mucoid material at birth. It lies almost in the centre of the intervertebral joint. But as age advances, the anterior part of the body of the vertebra grows much faster than the posterior part. Hence it ultimately lies strictly behind the centre. It forms a cushion between the vertebrae. There is a resultant compression which exerts evenly distributed hydrostatic pressure. The pressure within the nucleus is considerable.

The disc can be damaged by direct or indirect trauma. If the disc is healthy, it would need to be hit by a considerable force to be damaged. Even an impact enough to damage the body of a vertebra is not sufficient to damage a healthy disc. It has been calculated that a normal adult disc can withstand a compression force of 545 kg per square inch before rupturing, while less than 450 kg of pressure is enough to damage the vertebral body. In normal weight bearing, when a person is standing or sitting, the compression force is 45 kg. But it is estimated that it increases considerably, reaching upto 225 kg when a person is bending forward. In this position when a load of 30 kg is lifted by using only the spine while bending, the force increases upto about 450 kg, which is dangerously near the breaking limit. A weightlifter trained to lift with proper techniques can lift as much as 272 kg without any apparent

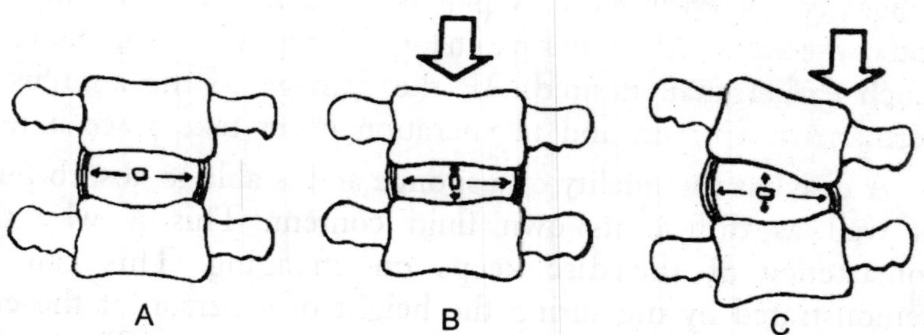

Fig. 3. Hydraulic (mobile) mechanism of the intervertebral disc. A. *Distribution of force on a normal disc;* B. *In a person carrying a heavy load on his head;* C. *While bending forwards.*

damage to the disc. This is why it is very important to learn the correct method of weightlifting. When the correct method is employed the weight is lifted with the help of the arm and leg leverage, and the weight is supported by the spine only when the person is erect. When a person lifts a weight, a small role is also played by the abdominal muscles, and part of the force is absorbed by the intra-abdominal structures. It is estimated that, while lifting, upto 30 per cent of the force is absorbed by these structures. This is why it is very important to have strong abdominal muscles in order to protect the lumbo-sacral spine. Exercising the abdominal muscles to make them strong is also important in case of lumbo-sacral pain.

When the disc has undergone degenerative changes, smaller weights may be sufficient to cause damage. So it is important to understand the degenerative changes of the disc to understand pain. It is also important to check or minimise degenerative changes as preventive measures.

The gelatinous properties of the nucleus depend upon its mucosaccarides which tend to break down with age. Imbibation of fluid diminishes, making the nucleus more rigid. The distance between the vertebral bodies diminishes; the annulus fibrosus bulges, growing weak at certain points. Under some circumstances and especially with trauma, the internal hydrostatic pressure

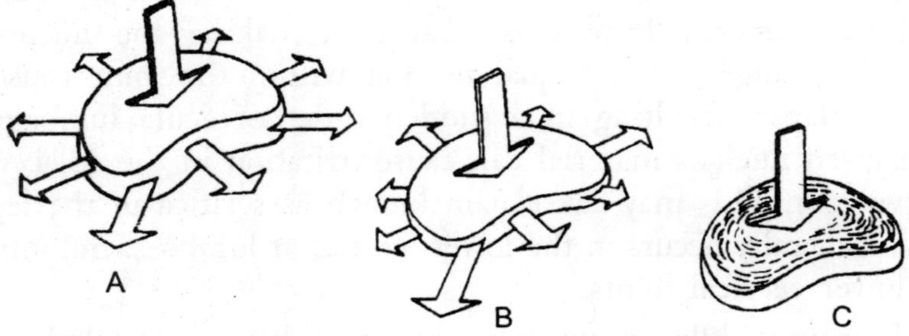

Fig. 4. Effect of pressure on the spinal disc at different ages. A. *Normal;* B. *With degeneration;* C. *With advanced degeneration. The problem of a slipped disc increases as the disc deteriorates with advancing age. A person with a slipped disc suffers from excruciating pain which can immobilise him.*

rises, and the weakened annulus gives way. The disc herniates or prolapses through the weakened annulus, which may, in turn, pass through the end plate. Symptomatology depends upon the location of the prolapse. The most susceptible area of the spine is the lower lumbar spine. It is here that spondylosis is most common. The intensity of the pain depends upon the sensitivity of the site of protrusion. Sometimes a fragment of the cartilage, generally in a degenerated disc, can break off and move inside the intervertebral joint, lodging against a sensitive area and causing pain. This pain may have a sudden onset. The broken fragments may consist of fibro-cartilage or nuclear tissue. The lumbar spine, however, is not the only part subjected to such pressures. For example, take the cervical spine. Here in spite of the smallness of the vertebrae, their bodies and facet joints support a large ball weighing approximately 5 kg — that is the man's head. The head is balanced over two small facets, small as nails, yet mobile in all directions. Some people can even carry a weight of upto 54 kg on their heads, entirely supported by the joints of the two upper cervical vertebrae.

After 20 years of age, degenerative changes start occurring, which may result in necrosis or breakage of the nucleus pulposus, and the softening and weakening of the nucleus fibrosus. Under these circumstances even a minor strain can cause internal derangement in the joint as the nucleus is displaced and the nucleus fibrosus is weakened, making the nucleus pulposus bulge out. Unequal tension within the joint causes disc-prolapse, resulting in a sudden onset of acute lumbago. Prolapsed nucleus material can cause irritation in the adjacent nerve root. This may cause pain known as sciatica in the leg. This generally occurs in the lower lumbar or lumbo-sacral joint or lower cervical joints.

During middle age, when degenerative changes start, bulging of the disc material may take place in any direction, producing a pull on the ligaments during weightbearing. A ligamentous pull lifts the periosteum from the margin of the body of the vertebrae. New bone formation takes place under this periosteal

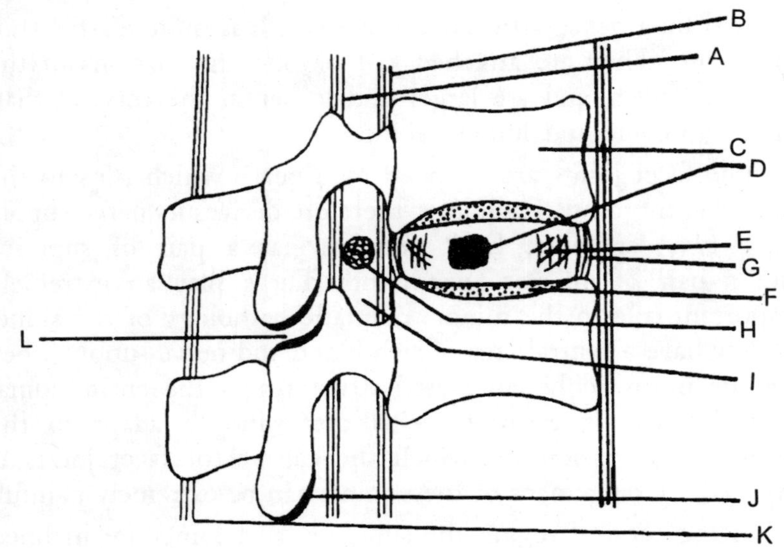

Fig. 5. The parts joining two vertebrae. A. *Ligamentum flavum;* B. *Posterior longitudinal ligament;* C. *Vertebral body;* D. *Nucleus pulposus;* E. *Annulus fibrosus;* F. *Cartilagenous plate;* G. *Intervertebral disc;* H. *Nerve root;* I. *Intervertebral foramen;* J. *Facet articular cartilage;* K. *Interspinous ligament;* L. *Facet joint.*

lift and in due course, osteophytes appear. These osteophytes, when viewed through an X-ray, are called osteoarthritic changes. They limit mobility. Ligaments also become hard by this age. Generally the osteophytes are thought to be responsible for pain, but in most cases they are not. This can be proved just by looking at a number of X-rays taken to reveal kidney stones in patients belonging to a middle or higher age group. Most of the time, the patients insist that they have never had a backache in their life.

The Posterior Joints

From a strictly anatomical point of view the posterior joints of the spine are the true joints of the spine. The extent and the variety of movement depends on the shape and direction of the facet joints (see Fig. 5). They determine the extent of movement and direction of a particular segment. These facet joints are covered by a dense articular capsule which is quite elastic, thin and loose. They are attached just beyond the margins of the articular facets, and are larger and looser in the cervical than in the thoracic and lumbar spine.

The facet joints are supplied by a nerve which runs to the two adjacent joints. Each joint therefore derives its nerve supply from two segments. Each vertebra has a pair of superior and a pair of inferior facet joints. These play an extremely important role in the minor traumatic pathology of the spine, as they have a central area of rich blood and nerve supply. They are the most richly innervated structures of the entire spinal column. This innervation helps the spine to adapt to the variation of tensions to which the capsule of facet joints is exposed. Derangement of these joints can be extremely painful.

In the cervical region the superior facet joints are inclined upwards at forty-five degrees. This helps in free flexion and extension of the neck. At this level usually, extension can be done more easily than flexion. Lateral bending and rotation are always combined.

In the thoracic region, the facet joints are more oblique, say, at an approximately sixty degrees inclination. In the upper part of the thoracic spine, movements are greatly restricted due to the direction of the facet joints and attachment of the ribs to the body of the vertebrae. Rotation at this level is of a greater range than flexion and extension. Lateral bending is restricted due to the ribs and the sternum.

Extension (backward bending) is freer in the lumbar spine. A considerable amount of side bending and a small amount of rotation can occur at this level.

Ligaments

The spine consists of a series of joints which are united from the second cervical to the first sacral by a number of ligaments. The vertebral bodies are united by anterior and posterior ligaments, and the posterior series of facet joints and neural arches are united by the ligamentum flavum (see Fig. 5).

The function of these and other ligaments is to hold the bone together and yet allow some calculated movements. The ligaments are elastic structures with an elastic limit. They remain healthy with intermittent stretching. Ligaments can be torn in two ways: sudden force and uninterrupted prolonged moderate stretching. This is why intermittent traction is more physiological than continuous sustained traction.

Anterior Longitudinal Ligament

A long and strong fibrous ligament runs on the anterior surface of the vertebrae. It is attached firmly to the disc and margins of the vertebral body, and loosely attached to the middle part of the body. It is wider at the level of the disc and narrower at the level of the body. A tear in any of the ligament fibres leads to haemorrhage, oedema and fibrin formation. If given sufficient time, the ligament becomes as strong as before, but if stretched too soon, it remains weak and repair is incomplete. The ligament may get elongated, making the joint hypermobile. When stretched continuously for prolonged periods, the ligament starts aching and its elasticity gets diminished.

Posterior Longitudinal Ligament

The posterior longitudinal ligament is attached to the posterior margin of the vertebral body within the vertebral canal. It forms a bridge over the body of the vertebrae and is attached firmly to the intervertebral disc and to the margins of the vertebral body. Thus it reinforces the disc posteriorly. This ligament plays an important role in disc protrusion. The resistance of the ligament helps to push the protrusion back again. The constant occurrence of lumbago in some persons may be caused because the protrusion is enlarged and pushed to the area of lesser resistance, thus producing unilateral sciatica pain. It is due to the posterior longitudinal ligament rupturing so completely, that the entire content of the intervertebral disc protrudes backwards and thus the *cauda equina* (lowermost roots of the spinal chord) is subjected to great pressure which may result in bilateral sciatica.

Muscles

There are quite a few muscles which act on the spine and help in its different movements. There are short muscles which act directly and long muscles which act indirectly and aid in the movements of the spine. They help to steady the spine. They produce extension, lateral bending and rotation.

Short muscles help to maintain the posture. They contract intermittently, and during an upright posture, there are slow spontaneous swaying movements. They help to extend the spine, along with the abdominal muscles. During flexion, the abdominal muscles also play a very active part. They help to initiate flexion and assist the short muscles in further flexion and control of it. It is surprising to know that in incomplete flexion, the short muscles are inactive and controlled by the spinal ligaments. Any imbalance and weakness of these muscles produces a deformity of the spine known as scoliosis.

Side bending is also helped by short muscles. They play a great role in mechanical vertebral pathology. A sudden, unexpected movement can produce a harmful distribution of the forces on the intervertebral joints. If certain parts are compressed or put into a traction beyond their capacity, they can damage the joint to a varying degree, depending on the force causing the painful muscle spasm. Synchronisation of muscular activity is more important than just increasing the strength of these muscles by various spinal exercises. This is why manipulation is an important therapeutic measure.

When the muscles are weak, the ligaments and joints are more strained, thus becoming more vulnerable. Generalised muscle weakness is also the cause of bad posture. Excessive powerful muscle contraction can also damage the bone: for instance, there can be a fracture of the kneecap due to contraction of the thigh muscles.

Intervertebral Foramen

The intervertebral foramen is a short canal lodged between contiguous vertebrae (see Fig. 5). It is ellipsoid in form. Its form changes with the mobility of the intervertebral joint. In the dorsal and lumbar spine it is directed laterally to the right and left. In the cervical spine it is directed slightly to the front, say by fifteen degrees, as compared to the dorsal or lumbar foramen. The canal is covered by a fibrous structure which is connected to the intervertebral disc and capsule of the posterior joints. Through it passes the spinal nerve which consists of a ventral root and a dorsal root. These appear to be united with each other in the canal, but when seen microscopically they are found to be separated. The dorsal root contains the spinal ganglion. Each spinal nerve, after coming out of the intervertebral foramen, has an offshoot of a small branch called a meningeal branch which re-enters the vertebral canal through the intervertebral foramen and ennervates the vertebral ligaments and blood vessels of the spinal chord.

The compression or irritation of elements contained in the intervertebral foramen may occur due to the degeneration of the disc, osteoarthritis of the intervertebral joints, posterior profusion of the disc, or rupture of the disc with herniation of the nucleus pulposus. This may cause pain, some muscular weakness, lumbago, sciatica and a diminished feeling all over the skin.

3
Adopting the Correct Posture

'My bed is so cosy, nice and soft. When I sleep I sink into it, I am in a dreamland and I feel wonderful and so fresh in the morning. I love my bed, it is so dear to me.' 'Disgusting!' said the osteopath.

'I have never played any game in my life. When I was young I entertained myself with novels and movies, or kept myself busy with my course books; I was a bookworm. When I got married, I hardly had any chance to participate in games. My house is well equipped with modern gadgets and amenities so that I hardly exert myself physically.' 'Frustrating!' said the osteopath.

'I was tall with good features, but since I was tall I could hardly hold myself erect. This was also due to the natural instinct of a teenaged girl. I gradually developed a habit of walking and sitting with a forward stoop. I cannot change it now.' 'So unmindful!' said the osteopath.

'If you go to Rajasthan, watch the ladies carrying a number of water pitchers on their heads. They walk miles and miles to bring water for the cooking and daily washing. It is a pleasure to see them walking. They walk so straight and their walk looks so very graceful.' 'Wonderful, it is healthy!' said the osteopath.

'Do you see boys making pyramid formations in a circus or on the streets of Bombay to bring down the pitcher hanging high and tied to a rope on *Janmashtami*? They make human pyramids, one boy over another, to reach the top to break the pitcher. Only a team of healthy and stout boys with straight backs can play this game and succeed.' 'It must be very interesting and so healthy!' said the osteopath.

'We live in a village and our work involves hard labour in the fields and at home. When we are young we go to the *akhada* to do *dand-baithak* and wrestling. We perspire, we rub mud on our bodies, we take a swim, we feel fresh and fine. We cannot afford thick mattresses, so we just spread a little rug on the ground and fall into a dreamless sleep, only waking up in the morning. We feel fine and energetic; we feel like pushing and punching somebody.' 'You have the healthiest habits in the world!' said the osteopath.

At the London College of Osteopathy, we used to hear an interesting story about a man called Frederick Matthias Alexander. He used to cure his patients of their aches and pain, only by teaching them how to stand and sit correctly and how to do different activities using the correct posture. He cured his patients just by correcting their posture! This may appear very surprising, but it is true. Osteopaths are very careful about the posture of their patients. They tell their patients how to correct their posture and do corrective exercises, so that once they are cured of their ailment, it will not recur. Medical men today are conscious of the role that posture plays in the etiology of different diseases.

It is very important to know how one should carry one's body. A humped back and vertebrae contracted together cause back pain. The neck sunk down on the chest causes stiffness in the neck, pain in the arm and headaches. When we stand erect, how many of us put equal pressure on both the legs? All the body weight is usually put on one leg, putting a constant strain on the pelvis and lumbar spine. Bad posture keeps our muscles tense.

How many teachers or parents are watchful of their child's posture? The correction of posture in a child is much easier than in grown-ups and elderly people. Healthy habits developed by a child help him right through his life. As parents or teachers, we should be conscious of how a child sits and if the posture is incorrect, we should point it out to him and take care to keep on correcting it. It is very important to see how a child sits, reads, writes, walks and plays.

Spinal curves are absent at birth and during the first few weeks of life, there is one continuous curve as the child is curled up in the womb. This primary curve undergoes changes as the child grows and lifts up his head, tries to sit, crawl, stand, walk and run. At the age of three months when the child tries to lift his head and look around, the upper secondary curve in the spine — from the first cervical to the first dorsal vertebrae — starts developing. By nine months when the child is able to sit, this curve is convex forward.

The lower spinal curve (lumbar) from the first lumbar to the fifth lumbar vertebrae appears between twelve to eighteen months when the child tries to walk. It is more prominent in females than in males.

The thoracic curve from the second to the twelfth thoracic vertebrae is concave forward. The pelvic curve from the lumbo-sacral joint to the coccyx faces downwards and forwards.

The primary thoracic kyphosis (bending forward at the thorax) present at birth is maintained; the cervical and lumbar lardosis (bending backward at the lower spine) are developed during the process of growth, so that man can assume an erect posture.

Biologically speaking the lumbar and cervical (neck) curves emerged after man acquired an erect posture during the evolution of human life.

Mechanically these curves are so constructed due to the structure of the vertebrae, that they are maintained even when we lie on the floor or an extremely hard bed. If these curves are excessive, they are a causative factor for different aches and pains. For example, the spinal joints most vulnerable to internal derangement are between the fifth and sixth cervical, and fourth

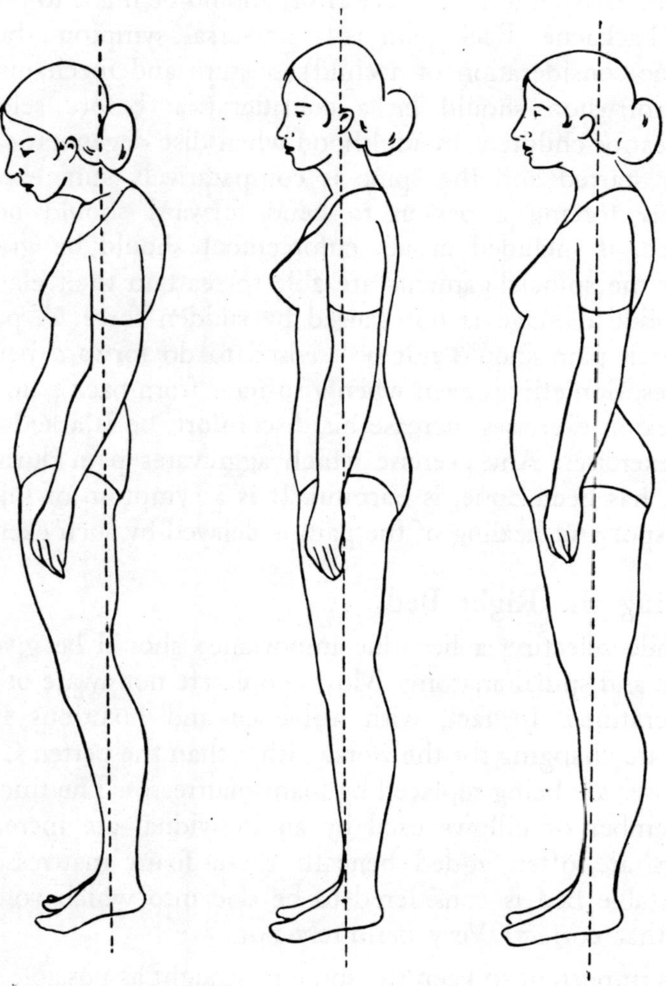

Fig. 6. Posture and pain. *The central sketch shows the correct posture. The other two sketches depict poor posture, which may lead to unequal pressure on the spinal joints and cause aches and pains.*

and fifth lumbar vertebrae — the area of the spine where the cervical and lumbar lardosis is most marked.

From early childhood every effort should be made to prevent future backache. Back pain is a universal symptom. So the aesthetic consideration of a child's posture and mechanism of disc protrusion should be a consideration before selecting exercises for children. In adulthood when disc degeneration has already started and the spine is comparatively stiff, exercises suddenly forcing a person to bend forward should not be included; if included at all, enforcement should be gradual, so that the spinal ligaments are able to reattain their elasticity and undue damage is not caused by sudden force. A patient with back pain should not be advised to do forward bending exercises. Sometimes even when a sufferer from back pain finds that flexion exercises increase his discomfort, he is asked to do these exercises. Any exercise which aggravates pain during or after it has been done, is harmful. It is a symptom of injuring a sore spot and healing of the pain is delayed by such exercises.

Selecting the Right Bed

While selecting a bed due importance should be given to posture and spinal anatomy. Most people are not aware of these considerations. In fact, with affluence and luxurious living, things are changing for the worse rather than the better. Cotton mattresses are being replaced by foam mattresses. The thickness and number of pillows used by an individual are increasing. Springs are often added beneath these foam mattresses. A comfortable bed is considered to be one into which you sink in. Is that correct? Very definitely not!

It is important to keep the spine as straight as possible while sitting, standing or doing any job. Equally important is to help the spine to remain as straight as possible while lying in bed, and even more so when you are suffering from back pain or neck pain.

Let us consider what a soft bed does to your spine. When you lie on a soft bed the heavier part of the body sinks deeper

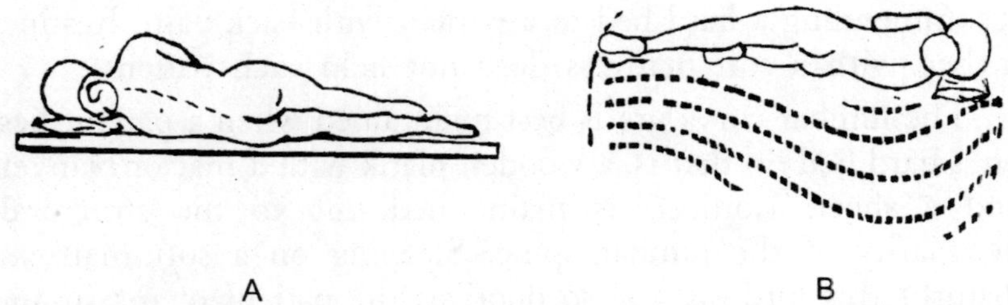

Fig. 7. Selecting a mattress. A. *Correct;* B. *Incorrect. The body sinks heavily when a person sleeps on such a mattress; this puts a heavy strain on the spine.*

into the bed, and the lighter part of your body stays up in bed, thus increasing the curvatures of the spine and putting a lot of undesired strain on it. Thick pillows worsen this situation. The thicker the pillow, the more you flex your cervical spine, which is again an unnatural strain.

The body has a great capacity to compensate. It compensates wrong posture for a long time. It does not complain till prolonged excesses are committed. However continuous prolonged strain gradually weakens the ligaments, leads to minor displacements in the intervertebral joints, and it is at this stage that the mechanism of the body, to compensate for undue strain, breaks down and we start feeling the pain.

The *brahmachari* or the pupil who went to his teacher and stayed with him in an *ashram* till he acquired sufficient knowledge and made himself fit for family life, was advised to sleep on the floor with a *kush* or rug made of grass. In *gurukuls* and even in the Banaras Hindu University founded by Madan Mohan Malaviya, students were provided with a wooden plank to sleep on.

A relaxation posture in yoga called *Shava asana* or Corpse pose is done by lying flat with the back on the floor with only a mat intervening. This *asana* is done to attain maximum relaxation of all parts of the body. Similarly hardness of the bed helps to maintain a straighter posture of the spine which is the normal posture — a posture of maximum relaxation and greater relief. This should be given due consideration while recommending a hard bed to a patient with back pain. Resting in bed with a soft mattress does not help such patients.

The lumbar curvature is best maintained when a patient lies on a hard bed — that is, a wooden plank with a mat or blanket and a sheet. Lordosis is maintained due to the structural peculiarity of the lumbar spine. Sleeping on a soft mattress disturbs this lordosis and so deprives the patient of maximum relief. Exercises are prescribed for patients with low back pain when their lumbar lordosis is obliterated. The lumbar curve can be compared to the arch of the foot, which is maintained by the peculiarity of the construction of the bones of the foot joint. This arch gives resilience to the foot and, due to the construction of the foot bones and the arches, provides it with strength and a springing action. The weight of the body is well distributed on the foot in order to bear the weight of the whole body and maintain its mobility.

The same is true about the construction of the lumbar and cervical vertebrae. When one lies flat on the floor without a mattress, the cervical and lumbar lordosis is in a posture of maximum relief and should be maintained in patients suffering from back pain and neck pain. Compare the quick fatigue you feel when you walk barefoot on the sand and the sand hampers the effective action of the foot arches. The same is true when you sleep on a thick foam mattress; it does not allow

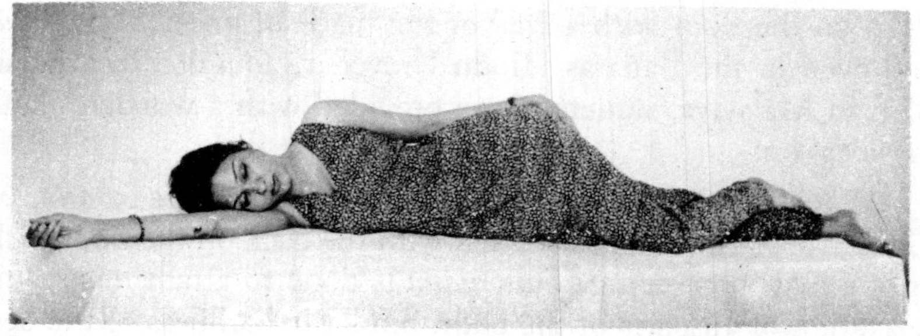

Fig. 8. Patient on a hard bed without a pillow. *This posture is good for low back pain and neck pain.*

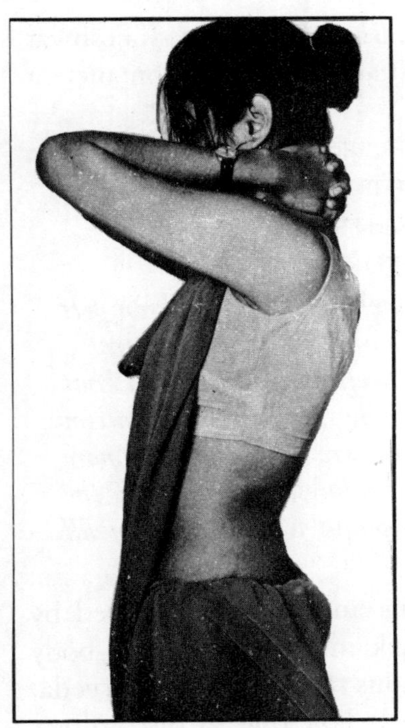

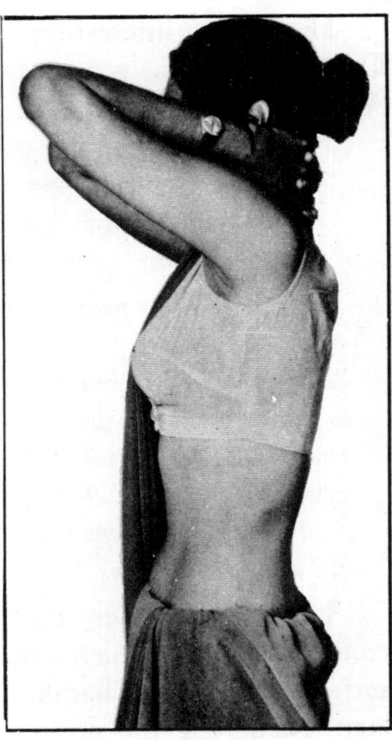

Fig. 9. Exercises for low back pain. A. *Stand erect and clasp your hands tightly behind your neck;* B. *Flatten the 'small' of your back by pushing the pelvis up and forward, so as to straighten the lumbar curve. This exercise can also be done by standing with your back against the wall and with feet flat on the floor.*

the lumbar lordosis to be maintained in a position of maximum comfort.

The best remedy for your tired back after a whole day's work is to lie down just for a few minutes with your back flat on the ground and you will feel relaxed.

Buddhists in ancient India lived in a monastery which consisted of a large hall with small rooms all around in the monastery. These rooms were often made by digging into big rocks, and stand to this date. Beds were also made by cutting into the rocks; these were for meditation and for the monks to sleep on.

There is an interesting *shloka* in *Bhav Prakash* by Rajeshwar Dutt Sashtri. This is one of the most authentic books on ancient Ayurveda.

सुशय्या शयनं ह्रदयं पुष्टिनिद्राधृतिप्रदम् ।
श्रमानिलहरं वृष्यं विपरोत मतोऽन्यथा ।।
त्रिदोषशमना खटवा तूलो वातकफापहा ।
भूश्य्या वृहणो वृष्या काष्टपट्टो तु वातहा ।।

To sleep on a proper bed stimulates the heart; a person gets good sleep, develops better patience, and his health improves. Sleeping on a bad bed has the opposite effect. Sleeping on a khat (a bed on four legs with tightened string top) helps rheumatism and a cough. He who sleeps on the bare earth will be more virile and strong. A wooden bed produces vatal, one of the dosas. He who sleeps on a wooden plank will be cured of all his aches and pains.

Ayurveda considers that all pains and aches are caused by *vata*, the energy which can get stuck in any part of the body and cause pain. Charaka, a famous teacher of Ayurveda, mentioned that 'the person who feels lazy due to discomforts in the body, and wants to sleep, should sleep on a somewhat hard bed' *(asukha shaiyya).*

When a person changes from a soft to a hard bed, he feels a little discomfort and slight stiffness in the beginning, but this phase passes off quickly and he later feels comfortable and relaxed.

A person who is healthy and does not have any back problem should have a bed with a solid base and a comfortable mattress, two to three inches thick. It can even be a foam mattress which is one inch thick. If there is a spring in the mattress, a wooden board should be placed on top of it and then a thin mattress. A patient with a spinal disc problem should be provided with a harder bed.

If pain and stiffness are felt after a night's sleep, it is an indication that the bed is faulty. During sleep, the muscles are relaxed and all the strain is tolerated by the ligaments. When these ligaments are stretched for a long time they start aching. This indicates that the bed is wrongly constructed and in spite of relaxing the spinal ligaments, it makes them taut, and pain is felt due to stretching of these ligaments.

Correcting Your Sitting Posture

Pain over the dorsal spine is very rarely due to a slipped disc. It is mostly due to the searing strain on the posterior ligaments of the spine, following a wrong posture. Due to the chronic habit of standing or sitting with a forward stoop, the patient develops a round back. This long-standing strain on the back weakens the spinal muscles. As the muscles are not able to take the strain, the strain passes on to the ligaments; and as the ligaments are continuously stretched for a long period, the body's compensation breaks and you start having back pain. When a patient has dorsal kyphosis, the site of the vertebrae placed at the summit of the dorsal curve feels most painful after fatigue. This pain may also radiate to the chest, shoulder and back. The cartilage of the disc is insensitive since it has no nerve supply and, therefore, the first sign of disc damage is due to the stretching of the supporting ligaments.

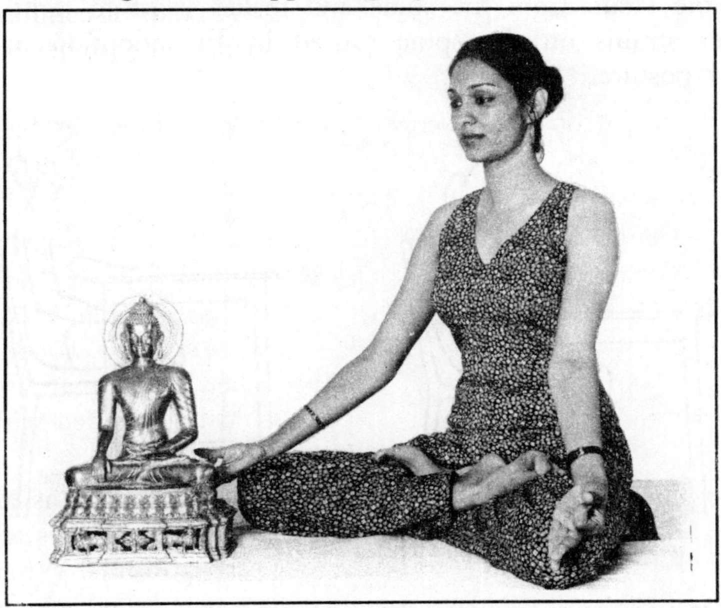

Fig. 10. *Yoga Mudra. A sitting posture (note the straight back) for meditation.*

The prolapsed disc may bulge and stretch the posterior ligament. A thin disc leads to narrowing of the space between the adjacent vertebrae of facets, with a consequent strain on the ligament which causes pain.

Have you observed the statues and paintings of Buddha at Ajanta and Ellora? Buddha is always shown sitting in *yoga mudra* with his spine straight. *Yoga mudra* is the sitting posture for meditation. This posture frees the body from any strain on the spine so that it does not hurt and divert the attention of the person who is meditating. This posture has to be maintained for hours and therefore, it should be comfortable, and free of any pain or strain.

Yoga asanas called posture exercises were developed in India in ancient times, and were practised for generations. *Asanas* are taught by Yoga teachers to patients suffering from back pain; they take the form of back extension exercises.

A simple set of exercises of *dand baithak* practised in the villages of India has a beneficial effect on the spine. It takes off the strain from the spine and makes it fit to fight the other strains on the spine caused by the adoption of an erect posture.

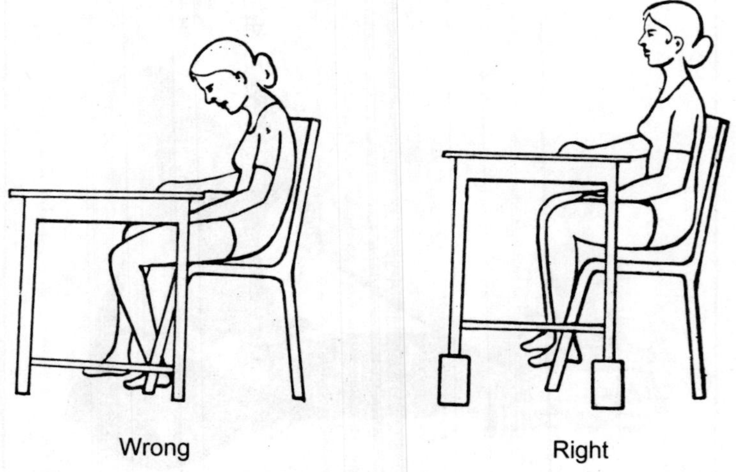

Fig. 11. Sitting posture. *Use a high table to avoid a stoop while at work.*

To sit slumping in a low chair puts considerable strain on the lower back. If the posture of sitting is not correct any measure to relieve the low back pain will not be effective. The patient should sit right at the back of the seat and then rest against the back of the chair. An ordinary office chair is much better than a sofa. If the cushion is not of a proper design, a small pillow may be placed behind the small of the back.

While designing furniture — be it a bed, kitchen shelves, or cupboards — keeping in mind the right posture is important. As an osteopath, I remember being paid a big fee for designing the chairs for the British Airways aircraft.

Strengthening Muscular Control

Exercises are needed to tone up the muscles and to maintain a good posture. Slack muscles lead to poor posture and undue strain is passed on to the ligaments. Eventually ligaments stretch and further abnormal mechanical strain produces still more symptoms.

Poor muscle tone is inevitable if the number and kind of exercises done are insufficient. A person with poor muscle tone is much more vulnerable to mechanical strain than one with a normal or muscular build.

An office worker, for example, whose spinal muscles are slack and weak due to his unstrenuous job, is much more vulnerable to strain or sprains if he tries to lift something heavy or do gardening. On the other hand, a person who does his exercises daily or participates in games has muscles which are in good shape. The following example will give a complete picture:

When a person is ill and completely inactive in bed, he loses the strength of the muscles at the rate of 7 per cent a day.

To increase the power of the muscles, exercises should be chosen wherein two-thirds of the maximum muscle strength is used.

To maintain the strength at the same level, one-third of the maximum strength should be used.

The power of the muscles decreases if only one-fifth or less of the maximum muscle power is used.

Increase in firmness and tone of the muscles is the indication of increase in muscle power. To acquire hypertrophy of their muscles, weightlifters and body builders exercise their muscles to a point of considerable fatigue. Hypertrophy of muscles is not necessary for healthy living.

The muscles should not be forced beyond a certain limit. If they are exercised beyond the tolerable muscle limit, they cease to contract in spite of maximum mental effort, and become inflamed, swollen and tender to touch. The subsequent contraction of muscles is painful for two to three days.

Mobility of the Spine

The intervertebral joints of the spine can be hypomobile (less mobile) or hypermobile (more mobile).

A hypermobile joint with elongated weak ligaments is more vulnerable to disc lesion. Hypermobility leads to impaired nutrition, and then degeneration and softening of the disc. In this case, as the supporting ligaments of the annulus fibrosus are weak, herniation of the disc is inevitable. Hypermobility also leads to injury and tearing of the ligaments, and when there

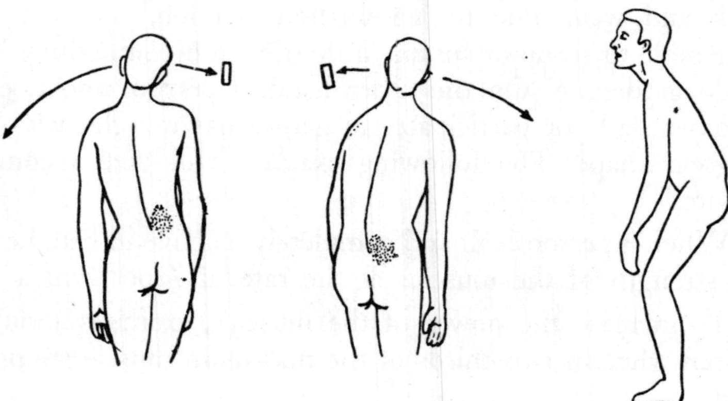

Fig. 12. *You may get acute pain after lifting a heavy object from the ground. Later this will force you to assume one of the postures as shown above.*

is a prolapsed disc, it takes much longer to heal, as giving support and rest to these joints is difficult.

A hypomobile spine has advantages over hypermobile joints. People with hypomobile spines are stocky and muscular. To have big muscles is not a disadvantage, but when such persons stop exercising, they suddenly become flabby. When exercise is not done, the muscles become poor in tone, and there is a likelihood of getting a mechanical strain.

The regulation of posture is governed largely through sensations emitted through the head. This is facilitated by the vestibule of the internal ear as well as by the nerve endings (called pacinian corpuscles) present in the ligaments of the cervical vertebrae.

An incorrect lifting posture is the reason why we sometimes get vertigo or giddiness due to disturbances in the upper cervical

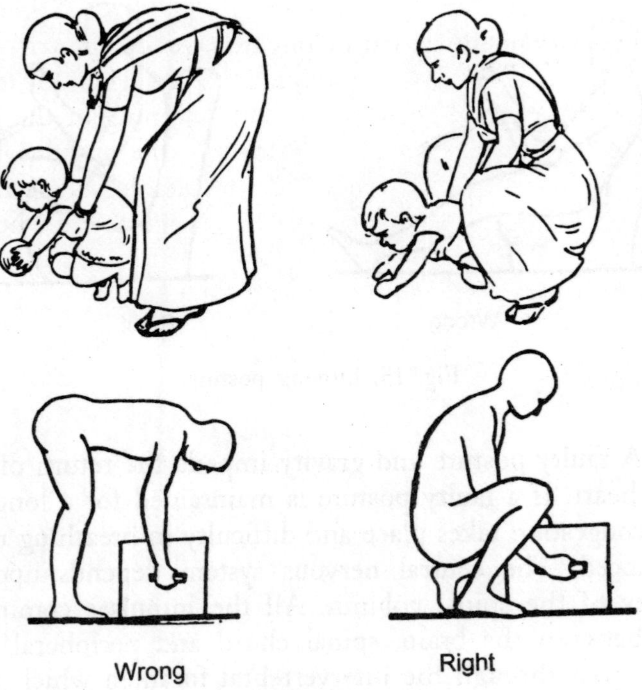

Fig. 13. Lifting posture.

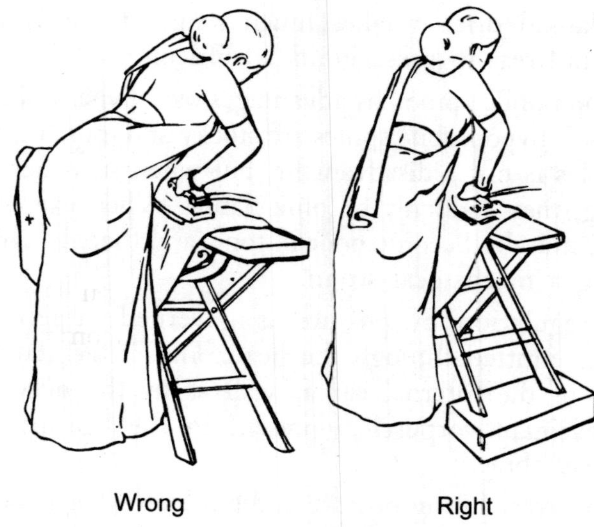

Fig. 14. Working posture.

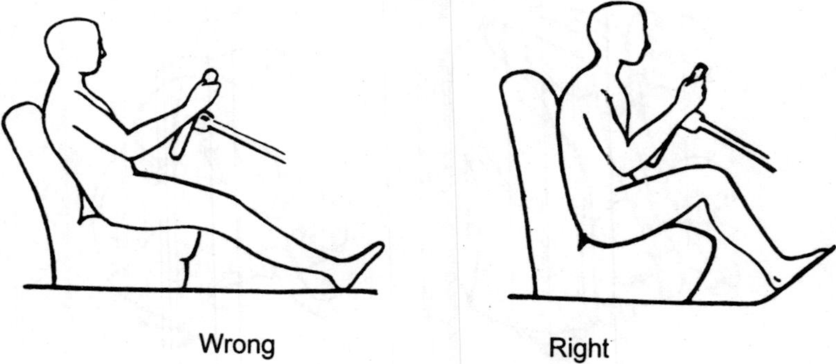

Fig. 15. Driving posture.

spine. A faulty posture and gravity impede the return of blood to the heart. If a faulty posture is maintained for a long time, blood congestion takes place and difficulty in breathing may be experienced. The central nervous system depends upon the integrity of the spinal column. All the impulses coming and going between the brain, spinal chord and peripheral nerves have to pass through the intervertebral foramen which can be very easily disturbed by a faulty posture, and can, in return, affect any part of the nervous system. Certain precautions must be taken to avoid a strain on the spine.

- When you want to lift something heavy from the ground or bathe a child, or make the bed, do not stoop; sit and lift the baby for a bath.
- Do not twist the body while turning, but rather change the position of your feet and turn. Just bending down and turning to one side is the worst movement you can make.
- Do regular back-extension exercises and abdominal exercises to keep up the tone of the muscles.

4
Manipulation of the Spine

You bend down to lift something heavy, perhaps your own child, and feel something 'go' in the small of your back. You feel an excruciating pain and cannot even get up.

One day, you feel pain and stiffness in your neck and you think that it may be due to an odd position your neck was in while sleeping.

Coming down the stairs you slip and sprain your ankle joint, or you open your mouth to yawn and cannot close it.

These pains start so suddenly and should have an equally short and effective treatment by which whatever has happened can be reversed. A lot of physiological changes occur in the pelvic region of the mother during childbirth. These may leave her with a low back pain. It was formerly thought that the cause of the pain was lack of proper care given to the mother after delivery. This is not true. Some re-adjustments which should take place of their own accord after the child is born, do not take place and the pain persists. Hence the cause of pain is purely mechanical.

Not only this, but a wrong method of sitting, standing, doing household work, or even a prolonged illness may leave you with a persistent back pain, sciatica, spondylosis, brachial neuralgia, headache, insomnia or even dysmenorrhoea.

There are innumerable problems which can be narrated one after another, and which are so common. What are the possibilities for their cure and what possible remedies can you get for them? The pain may clear in a few days and you may think it was a simple sprain or myalgic pain. Or when it is unbearable, you may land in hospital where a lot of investigations are conducted and X-rays taken. You may be told that the pain is due to a slipped disc or spondylosis.

You are probably advised to take complete bedrest for a few weeks, undergo diathermy (which will emit heat to your deep-seated joint) or massage, continuous or intermittent traction, wear a collar or belt, take medication, use applications, do remedial exercises or try out some other treatment.

There is a possibility of getting cured. But it is also probable that in spite of devoting a lot of time, undergoing torturous treatment and heavy expenses, the pain persists.

Ultimately you are told by a specialist or a consultant, 'You are going to have this pain throughout your life; this pain will not go and you should learn to live with it.' You may also be advised to have disc surgery without any assurance about the result. And even if you are cured following the operation, you will have a weak back and will live the rest of your life, taking a lot of precautions and observing many dos and don'ts.

Many patients end up going to a healer who may hang them upside down and tie their ankles to the roof, for half an hour every day, day after day. Some may be given electric shocks. In other cases red hot iron rods may be pressed over the area of pain. Some patients even resort to witchcraft, faith healers, *sadhus* and *mullas*. They may be asked to wear a copper bracelet, or they may go to a bone setter and get cured by sheer luck. If they are wise, they will resort to vertebral manipulation.

After my medical graduation I joined the Central Institute of Orthopaedics, New Delhi, one of the most reputed orthopaedic institutes in the country. Patients with various types of pain came in large numbers and in spite of the best facilities of diagnosis and treatment, we did not seem to be helping them much. Week after week, month after month ... the treatment seemed to be unending in quite a few cases. While we were so effective in the treatment of fractured bones and other ailments, I kept wondering why we could not help patients with chronic aches and pains. I consulted my orthopaedic books to find that manipulation was mentioned as one form of treatment. Why were we not using it? I tried to question my teachers but they could not give me a satisfactory answer. I then decided to go to England to become an osteopath.

Manipulation is an art, a science and a philosophy. Manipulation is sometimes called orthopaedic medicine or *finger surgery* by medical practitioners.

Manipulation is one of the oldest techniques used for healing different ailments of the body. Bone-setters have been known to exist since olden days in almost all parts of the world. However they seem to have confined themselves to fracture cases, and used a few manipulative manoeuvres. Manipulation has been successful in a few cases though without carrying out any diagnosis. It was mostly done by lay persons without any knowledge of human physiology and pathology.

Hippocrates, the father of medicine, used to manipulate the spines and joints of his patients. A table used by him for this purpose is still preserved at the Welcome Historical Museum, London.

Sushruta, the famous surgeon of ancient India, used to manipulate many of his patients; he describes this in his *Asthichikitsa* (Bone Treatment).

This method of treatment is not readily accepted by modern medical men. Manipulation attracts criticism, misconception and scepticism, and rightly so, as it has mostly been done by lay manipulators. In the absence of knowledge of pathology, grievous injuries may be caused to patients. It has often been referred to in the following manner: 'A brutal and blind treatment ...' 'A dangerous form of psychological treatment ...' 'An occasional good result does not compensate for the accidents it can produce....' Often these criticisms stem from people who have not participated in a well-conducted manipulation session. This criticism is, however, now dying out, since many medically qualified people are being drawn towards it. It is now being built upon a sound scientific base and is the main therapeutic measure used by orthopaedic surgeons abroad and by a few in India as well.

Many appreciative comments have also been coming forward: 'Results are astonishing ...' 'It shortens the period of recovery and protects a patient from prolonged agony and mental apathy ...' 'It avoids many an unnecessary operation ....'

With the development of the osteopathic profession and hospitals, colleges and research centres, manipulation has become more accurate and scientific. Several orthopaedic surgeons abroad manipulate each and every case, and resort to an operation only when manipulation fails. There are signs of increased respectability being given to manipulation as a therapeutic measure. If a patient wants to recover fast, the physician is also equally anxious to cure his patient as fast as he can. This gives him great work satisfaction.

When I got admission to the London College of Osteopathy in September 1966, most of my colleagues were British general practitioners who had 10-15 years of lucrative general practice behind them. They were not happy with their results; sometimes they did not know how to help their patients. After hearing about manipulative treatment, they tried to learn one or two techniques from a friendly osteopath, used them casually on their patients and were so happy and surprised at the results that many of them decided to leave their practice, learn manipulation more thoroughly and in greater detail, and after completion of the course, and convinced of its efficacy, settled into full-time manipulative practice. At first it seemed unbelievable to me that patients could improve so much with the use of one's hands. How right was the saying that a certain physician had 'fame in his hands!' His mere touch was enough to cure! This may have been an exaggeration, but the importance of hands cannot be denied, especially for a manipulative physician. A physician's hands convey compassion and understanding — more so those of an osteopath who makes use of his hands more than any other physician.

Susceptibility of the Spine to Pain

Why is the spine so susceptible to pain? The answer lies in man's aquisition of an erect posture. During the process of evolution, man became a biped from a quadruped. When walking on four feet, the spine was supported by the two hands and feet. It never had to bear the flexion strain as it had no need to bend forward, being supported by the feet.

When man assumed an erect posture, the compression and flexion strains were added to the spine, for which it was not designed. Worst of all, each pair of nerves emerged from the weakest portion of the spine — that is, the intervertebral joints. Moreover each joint contained a disc (except the two uppermost) — a ring of fibro-cartilage with a pulpy centre, and a nucleus pulposus, adding further to the spinal weakness.

The physical and mechanical factors which influence the body are complex entities. Apart from environmental and inherent factors, gravity, pressure, weight, elasticity, leverage, movement, and so on, also play a great role.

The normal contraction of muscles counteracts gravity, the elasticity of ligaments allows the joints to move, while countless mechanical forces act and interact with each other. This is the realm of applied mechanics of the human body. The spine is vulnerable even to normal mechanical stress. This abnormal stress due to bad posture, or an abnormal strain due to a jerk, twist or strain, or a fall can produce a mechanical disturbance in the spine known as an osteopathic lesion.

Osteopathic Lesion

An osteopathic lesion is a condition of impaired mobility in an intervertebral joint, in which there may or may not be an altered positional relationship of the adjacent vertebrae. When there is restriction of movement it is always within full range of movement. It can be caused by:

- A specific injury, a fall, twist, strain, athletic strains, lifting heavy objects;
- A faulty posture, occupational and environmental hazards, habit or hereditary weakness;
- A lesion present elsewhere;
- Reflex due to certain infections like cold, influenza, pneumonia, draughts, exposure, abuse or excessive use of any part of the body

An osteopathic lesion is not as pronounced as dislocation. A lesion causes pressure on the nerves, altered blood circulation, oedema, tissue changes, muscle spasms. In the case of a chronic lesion, the adjacent joints sometimes become hypermobile and compensate for the restricted movement. This restricted movement at a particular intervertebral joint is difficult to diagnose, since the movement at these intervertebral joints is very small individually. But in combination with others, it is very marked. So if there is a little restriction at one or two intervertebral joints, it may not be noted in certain cases and this is why it produces a lot of difficulty in diagnosis during the clinical examination. There should be an osteopathic examination to detect this condition.

Apart from a clinical examination, osteopaths depend on palpatory diagnosis: the feel of the tissue, the feel of the muscle, the feel of the movements at the intervertebral joint. To be familiar with this type of feel and appreciate and distinguish the variation in different patients by a physician who is not trained osteopathically, is difficult. Clear demonstrations of these changes by a measuring gauge or a clear distinction and demarcation is not possible. This is also one of the causes due to which physicians look at their osteopathic colleagues with scepticism.

Osteopaths have to use their hands a lot in diagnosis and treatment. Their sense of touch improves with constant use, the feel becoming more refined. They are able to distinguish even a small tissue change, muscle spasm, difference in the warmth of the area; even the difference in mobility or restriction of movement with the help of their fingers, with the help of their sense of touch. They try to 'see' through their fingers, they have 'thinking' fingers. Blind men, for instance, have a much more refined sense of touch and a much sharper feel. This refinement comes through constant use.

At the London College of Osteopathy, we were each handed a six-pence coin. We were told to keep it in our pockets, and feel it constantly with our fingers. We were asked to try and locate the queen's crown, the nose, the ears — to just feel and keep on feeling so as to be able to distinguish them easily. A student in medical college is raw; he has to build upon the clinical knowledge he acquires at college to become a better physician or surgeon. So it is with an osteopath. When an osteopath comes out of an osteopathic college, he has only a base. With the constant use of his fingers and his clinical sense, the precision of his judgement makes him a better osteopath.

Every doctor cannot be a good surgeon; similarly, everybody cannot become a good osteopath. This is why osteopathy has been called an art. Everybody cannot be a master of the sitar or violin. It calls for a natural instinct and inherent qualities, besides rigorous training.

Osteopathic treatment cannot be prescribed like medicine three times a day. An osteopath cannot say, 'Take traction for 15 minutes every day with a fifteen-pound weight for ten days, or take diathermy for 10 minutes every alternate day for ten days.' It is difficult to prescribe the amount of force to be applied or the sequence of manoeuvres. Having a comprehensive grasp of the subject, osteopaths diagnose the disease as they go on with the examination and programme their techniques accordingly. The same thing is repeated at every visit of the patient. Osteopathy is not just manipulation. It includes understanding the mechanical problem, the patient, the contributory factors, and then adapting the technique at the time of treatment to the patient.

A few techniques can definitely be taught to general practitioners or physiotherapists, and applying them will definitely give them a certain amount of success. Who can deny the fact that bone-setters are sometimes successful? They have learnt a few manoeuvres as a family tradition and use them on patients.

The scope of osteopathy is much wider. An osteopath's hands are his instruments. Hands can console, communicate, inspire hope, give strong suggestions and induce confidence in the patient. The doctor who gives treatment with his hands induces much more confidence in a patient than when the same is done by a third person or by a technician using the best of techniques.

In recent years a big advance has been made by the medical profession in using manipulation as a therapeutic measure. Way back in 1945, Cyriax made it known that back pain, sciatica, cervical spondylosis and brachial neuralgia were due to a slipped disc. Since then manipulative treatment has obtained a firm footing in the medical world. The most effective treatment for a slipped disc or protrusion of the intervertebral disc now is to slip it back to its normal position. This is what osteopaths aim at. Most orthopaedic surgeons use manipulation on their patients. Treating these cases with heat, liniment, muscle relaxants and pain killers implies sticking to the old medical belief which considered the cause of pain to be muscular, and so named it fibrositis or myositis.

If the number of disc operations being performed five years ago was one hundred, these have now been reduced to about five. How has this figure fallen so drastically? The answer lies in manipulation. Surgeons have begun to understand better the futility and poor results of disc surgery. Surgery can lead to neurological damage.

Osteopathy recognises the structural abnormality of the spine. It aims to normalise the mechanical defects and when this is not possible, it tries to make the body adapt itself to the structural weakness. Structural abnormality has an adverse effect on the harmony and efficiency of the body. These faults sometimes persist long enough for diseases to appear. The body is constantly trying to restore itself to normalcy, and thus to normal health. A spontaneous restoration to good health after an accident or illness is the rule. Most fractures unite whether we help nature or not, but the result is functionally better, if during the repair, we splint the bone into normal alignment. It should be our aim to help nature as much as we can by removing mechanical hindrances.

When we manipulate the spine, we are not so concerned about putting the bone back into place, as with removing mechanical hindrances, if any, and the restoration of normal movements in the affected joints. Our effort does not embrace the static structural problem. We are more concerned about the dynamic structural problem. Mechanical disturbances can adversely affect the body in the following way:

1. Irritation or compression of nerves can lead to pain, and increase or decrease conduction in the nerves.

2. Irritation or blocking of blood vessels can lead to initial ischaemia (reduction of blood supply to parts of the body), and later, congestion of blood and oedema.

3. Abnormal compression of a bone can lead to sclerosis or alteration in its shape.

4. Abnormal leverage on joints can lead to weakness or tearing of ligaments, damage to cartilage — both inside and outside the joint, and irritation of the synovial membrane.

When mechanical adjustment is done, it stops deterioration of the bone and tries to normalise abnormalities as far as possible.

Lord Brain (1963) maintained that the chief reason for manipulation was to reduce an intra-articular displacement.

Since cervical spondylosis is secondary to the changes in the disc symptoms, in the early stages it stems mainly from a minor degree of disc protrusion. We have clear confirmation that prophylaxis and the treatment of choice in these cases is manipulative reduction. It is the first treatment to be considered unless some contraindication exists.

Myrin (1967) compared a series of cases of pain in the lower back treated by conventional methods (rest in bed, physiotherapy, corsetry, and so on) and manipulation, and his results were tabulated as follows:

Effectiveness of Spine Manipulation

	RELIEF			
Treatment	*Total*	*Moderate*	*Slight*	*None*
Conventional	4%	21%	49%	26%
Manipulative	23.5%	23.5%	53%	0%

According to the *Sunday Citizen* of June 20, 1975, an American firm compared the effect of manipulative treatment of backache for 15 months with that of traditional treatment given for 15 months earlier. They found that the total days lost from work dropped from 1,203 to 119.

Disorders causing neck stiffness, arm pain, sciatica, and so on, can be usually recognised for their true nature. However, when spinal disorders occur in the area where they cause remote symptoms resembling heart disease or gastro-intestinal disease, then the situation becomes difficult. It is disastrous when a life-threatening disease goes unrecognised. But it is equally disastrous to be given a false diagnosis of heart disease or lung disease or some other serious affliction, when in reality the cause lies in the accessible and treatable condition of the spine.

We are apt to label a normal heart as diseased because of the failure to understand the mimicking effect of the mechanical disorder of the musculo-skeletal system. This problem is a serious one and is one of the main concerns of the osteopathic profession. In fact the differential diagnosis of pain is one of the main concerns of the medical profession. To ignore the fact that pain in a remote area may be caused due to a disturbance in the musculo-skeletal system will be to ignore a major fact of medicine. Doctors of medicine are beginning to write articles and books on this finding.

Ordinary backaches and recurrent headaches are annoying but do not provoke fear. It has been determined that a common cause of headache is the disorder of the cervical spine. It is very important that any mechanical disorder of the cervical spine should be recognised and treated as a common cause of headache.

Symptoms often appear at a distance from the lesion, as for example:

- Disease of the gall bladder can cause pain in the right shoulder.
- Disease of the heart can cause pain in the left shoulder.
- Disease of the kidney can cause pain in the loin.
- Disease of the stomach can cause pain in the back between the shoulder blades.

If this is possible why it should not work the other way around too? Our nervous system is not a one-way street. It conveys impulses from the inside of the body outwards and from the surface of the body inwards. This fact has long been known but never appreciated.

Disturbances affecting the surface of the body skin, muscles, ligaments and tendons may simulate diseases of the body organs. So the mimicking effect of these disturbances, while making a diagnosis of a certain disease, should definitely be given consideration.

A patient with disorders of the musculo-skeletal system is often treated as a 'neurotic'. This sort of miscalculation is enough to cause neurosis. There are cases on record, where electric shock treatment has been given for a 'neurotic-back' patient; this was later corrected by osteopathic manipulative treatment.

The sixty per cent of the body mass which comprises our musculo-skeletal system should be given due consideration in any diagnosis.

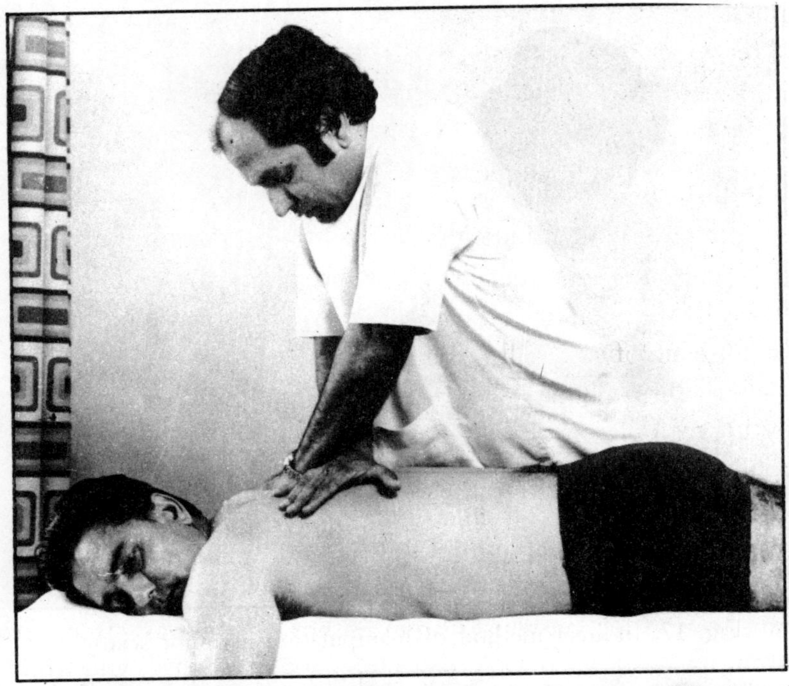

Fig. 16. Direct method of manipulation used for upper back pain.

Manipulation can be done in four ways:

Direct. The method of applying direct pressure is used on the spine itself (Fig. 16). This manoeuvre is generally used by chiropractors. Pressure is applied by the heel of the hands. The exact force is short and sharp. It is mostly applied at a level of transverse processes. It necessitates a strong pressure which cannot be graded. It is often unpleasant and sometimes painful, and often has limited use.

Indirect. The manipulations are done indirectly through levers formed by the hands, shoulder, pelvis and legs (Fig. 17). No pressure is put directly on the spine. The osteopath manipulates in all directions, through every vertebra, and the strength used is always possible to grade. The patient is properly positioned. This helps the operator to execute measured mobilisation and this movement can be repeated. This manoeuvre is mostly painless. A very mild push, a slight jerk, a little passive

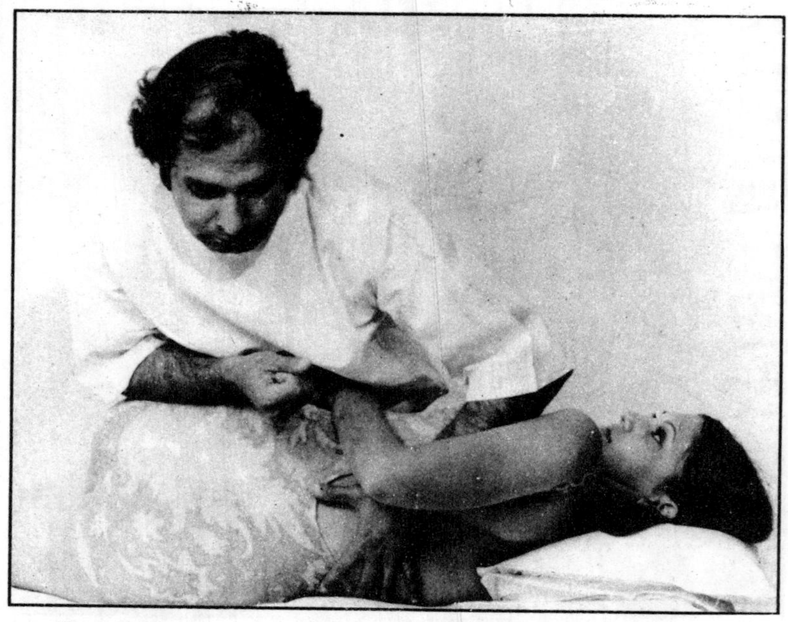

Fig. 17. Indirect method of manipulation used for sciatica.

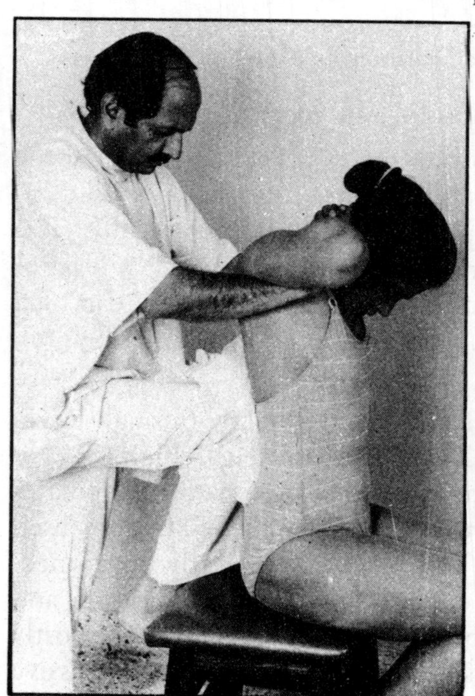

movement — all bring great relief.

Semi-Indirect. This is applied for higher precision in different regions of the spine. Direct pressure is applied to the manipulated segment with the help of the hand, knee or chest (Fig. 18). Manipulation is accomplished by a sudden movement of a distant part. Counter-pressure is applied by the hand, knee or chest.

Fig. 18. Semi-indirect method of manipulation for low back pain.

Constant Pressure. This is used for the cranial region. It is applied in a particular direction depending on the articulation of the cranial bones (Fig. 19). There is no possibility of using leverage as the shape of the skull does not allow it.

When bones are moved while manipulating, a click by a palpating hand is sometimes audible even from a distance. This is not due to the disc being pushed back into position. It is the sound of separation of the two surfaces in a particular joint. The sound originating from the disc is a very soft one; it is generally not audible but definitely palpable.

Manipulation often needs to be repeated in a long-standing case at certain intervals — generally of one week. This provides a complete opportunity for the repair and healing process of the torn fibrosis and intervertebral joints which have moved slightly. The time interval of one week may be shortened or prolonged in selective cases.

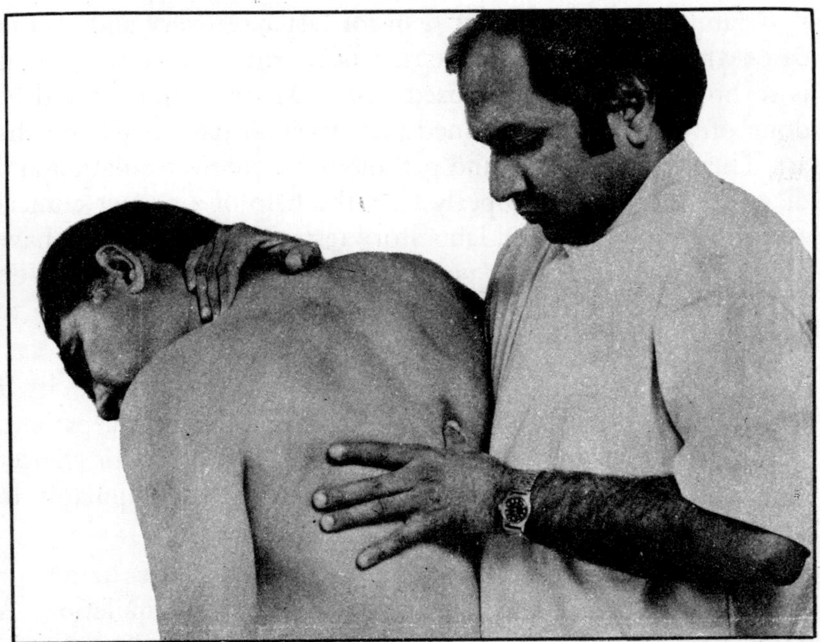

Fig. 19. The constant pressure method of manipulation used for localised pain in the middle back.

In a disordered intervertebral joint, the muscles and ligaments get shortened and fibrosis takes place. Manipulation is done to remove the fibrosis and to position mal-positioned bones, ligaments and muscles. This manoeuvre quite often needs to be repeated. Generally, relief starts from the very first treatment. Occasionally, two to three treatments are required before relief is felt.

No fixed rule can be laid down about the number of times treatment may be needed for a particular case. Each case is subject to individual assessment.

An osteopath generally does manipulation without anaesthesia. Here the patient's own resistance also comes into play and helps to avoid over-manipulation of the joint. A mild push, a very slight jerk or even a little passive movement is far more helpful than great force or a loud noise.

Precautions

Manipulation is of great help for faster recovery and also in cases which are not amenable to other forms of treatment. This is so however, only if it is used wisely. Manipulation should be done only by properly trained persons who have mastered the art. They should understand pathology before manipulating and diagnose the disease properly with the help of a proper clinical examination, X-rays and laboratory tests. It is necessary to have a good X-ray picture. A poorly taken X-ray may miss out on a fracture of a vertebra which is an absolute contraindication to manipulation.

The actual pathology of the spine where the bone itself is involved must be understood before manipulating a patient. Manipulating a case of tuberculosis of the spine or cancer or a tumour of the spinal chord may land a manipulator in trouble.

A patient suffering from incontinence of urine or uncontrolled bowel action is not a case for manipulation. A patient who has severe pain and cannot move in bed should not be manipulated till the pain has subsided considerably through bedrest and other therapeutic methods. In fact 1 to 2 weeks should be allowed to pass before manipulative treatment is given.

Manipulative manoeuvres also differ in different cases. In one case, forceful manipulation may be needed but in another, mild manipulation may do. It is always better to adopt a milder manoeuvre than a forceful one. Manipulation should also be tried in cases where it cannot cure completely, but can provide considerable relief. Cases of old-standing osteoarthritis of the knee and spine (ankylosing spondylitis or bamboo spine) can get considerable relief by this method. Some cases respond in a very short time, others take longer. A patient who has been suffering for a long time takes a longer time to heal than a person whose pain is of a shorter duration. In old cases, where there is disuse of a particular limb as a result of pain, there may be muscle wasting or reduction in girth, but the patient recovers as the pain disappears and normal use of the limbs is resumed.

Manipulation should not be repeated too often, and should not be carried out till improvement continues after the first treatment. Ideally, it should not be repeated without a gap of a week or fortnight, or till considerable recovery has taken place. A few patients need maintenance manipulation twice or thrice a year, so that recurrence of the disease does not take place, specially in cases of postural strain.

Many patients with a prolapsed disc in the lumbar spine feel better while walking and standing rather than sitting. They are advised to maintain a horizontal or vertical position and to avoid half-lying or sitting for long periods.

Prolonged bedrest is not desirable; it does not accelerate recovery and tends to weaken the general musculature. The morale of the patient also reaches a low ebb.

Activities which accentuate the pain should be avoided, especially those activities following which pain is accentuated. This is an indication that the nerve root has been irritated and has got inflamed due to activity.

A corset (belt) can be worn for short periods. It reduces the risk of irritation to the nerve root and reminds the patient to take care, thereby helping to avoid recurrence of the problem. If it is worn for a longer time, however, the muscles become weak and wasted. Thereafter, taking off the corset becomes difficult. After recovery, the patient should be encouraged to do certain exercises to strengthen the muscles and to develop a natural corset of his own muscles, thereby discarding the artificial one as soon as possible.

Manipulation is safe and complications do not occur if due precautions are taken, and unnecessary force is not applied. An occasional accident cannot be completely ruled out. But merely for this reason it is neither fair nor wise to condemn manipulation.

If an occasional death under anaesthesia, a fatal haemorrhage or surgical shock, or failure of surgical techniques led to total condemnation of surgery, then the human race would be worse off. Similarly it is unwise to condemn all manipulations, simply because on one or two occasions, the patient's condition has worsened. The fault lies with the manipulator and not with manipulation!

5
Curing Headaches and Migraine

A headache is a common problem today. Who does not get a headache? An executive, a philosopher, a scientist, a business magnate, a clerk, a housewife, a student — everybody, at sometime or other, is afflicted by a headache! It has no professional or age barriers.

Women suffer more than men. The reason may well be premenstrual migraines during puberty. These get worse as the years roll by, and are cured only by menopause. Contraceptives are known to cause headaches in some women and cure them in others. Headaches may become less frequent in pregnancy.

In fact, a headache is not a killing disease, but its attack is so intense that all the nerves in the skull start throbbing due to great pressure.

A lot of research has been done to find out the cause of headaches. What is a headache? Is it an allergic disease caused by something we eat or breathe? Has it any relation to our posture, incorrect way of sitting, standing or working? Is it a product of tension in our day-to-day life, a way to relieve frustration? Or is it due to some mechanical problem in the neck or head itself?

In the 5th century, it was thought that a headache was due to a severe chill, exposure to sunlight, or even fatigue. In the 11th century, it was thought that it occurred after having cold things in our food. According to Tissort (1784), vomiting often concluded an attack. He also suggested that a reflex irritation of the gastric nerves resulted in an attack of migraine. Living (1873) said that a headache was related to asthma and a convulsive state. Rilay (1932) suggested that it occurred when noxious vapour entered the cerebral blood vessels. According to another opinion, it occured due to eye strain. A few researchers concluded that it was due to adhesions of the cerebral membranes and formation of excessive cerebro-spinal fluid. Disorders of the ovaries and thyroid were also thought to cause migraines. Emotional problems were also attributed to headaches — for instance, a difficult father-and-son relationship in business, tough competition, a tense situation in the family, a hard struggle to get oneself established .... Apart from this, certain foods were found to cause headaches: chocolate, cheese, fruits, alcohol, fatty fried foods, tea, coffee, sea food, pork and many more.

Remedies

The long series of researches in this direction have shown that the human race has suffered a lot from headaches and though thousands of remedies have been prescribed, they have only succeeded in providing temporary relief. Many migraine clinics and foundations have spent millions of rupees to find a remedy which will bring permanent relief. These efforts are akin to ploughing in the sand! How long have we to live with such strong medications which produce side-effects in other systems of our body? After using a particular medicine for a long time, it loses its effectiveness anyway.

Sometimes, while suffering from a headache, a striking idea, solution or news gets rid of the headache and the patient becomes normal again. During a battle, General Ulysses S. Grant was seized with an attack of migraine. The limping general received the good news that his enemy was ready to surrender. Ulysses sprang to his feet at this glad news, and his headache vanished miraculously.

Many victims change their environment, take to the Himalayas, Tibet or Somaliland, go from the highest altitude to the lowest, from the wettest to the driest, experiencing a new climate, food and cultural changes but the migraine remains, because they carry their personal environment with them.

Headache of Cervical Origin

Frequently, a chronic headache resistant to treatment is due to a disorder of the cervical spine, which may be cured by manipulation. Certain mechanical changes in the cervical spine may cause an intermittent or a continuous headache. These changes respond well to manipulation. The pain can spring from the neck. Some people do not believe in the possibility that pain can radiate from the neck to the head.

An experiment was carried out by Kellgreen. A concentrated saline solution was injected in the area where the cervical spine first joins with the head, producing tenderness and headache in the forehead region. This proved a connection between the neck and the forehead.

Important changes have been found in the cervical spine in cases of headaches. These relate to disturbances in the lumin of the vertebral artery which passes through the transverse process of the cervical vertebrae and supplies blood to the brain.

Sometimes the therapeutic effect of cervical manipulation helps us to confirm whether a particular headache is of cervical origin.

Sometimes a headache is produced by the head being kept in a certain position; keeping it in the opposite direction relieves the headache. Sometimes manual traction at the neck relieves the headache. These are indications that headaches may be of cervical origin, and manipulation succeeds.

Embryologically, the head and the first and second cervical vertebrae are formed by the first and second cervical segment.

As they originate from the same segments they ought to

have some relationship between them. So any abnormality at the level of the first and second cervical vertebrae can give rise to pain in any part of the head, the temple and the forehead. As it happens elsewhere, local pain at the level of the cervical vertebrae may be completely absent and the patient may complain only of a headache.

This type of headache may come on while waking up in the morning. It may be felt in the back of the head or the front of the head, or may be only in the forehead. This begins to ease after some hours and is much better by mid-day. The patient is free from headache till the next morning. As the years pass

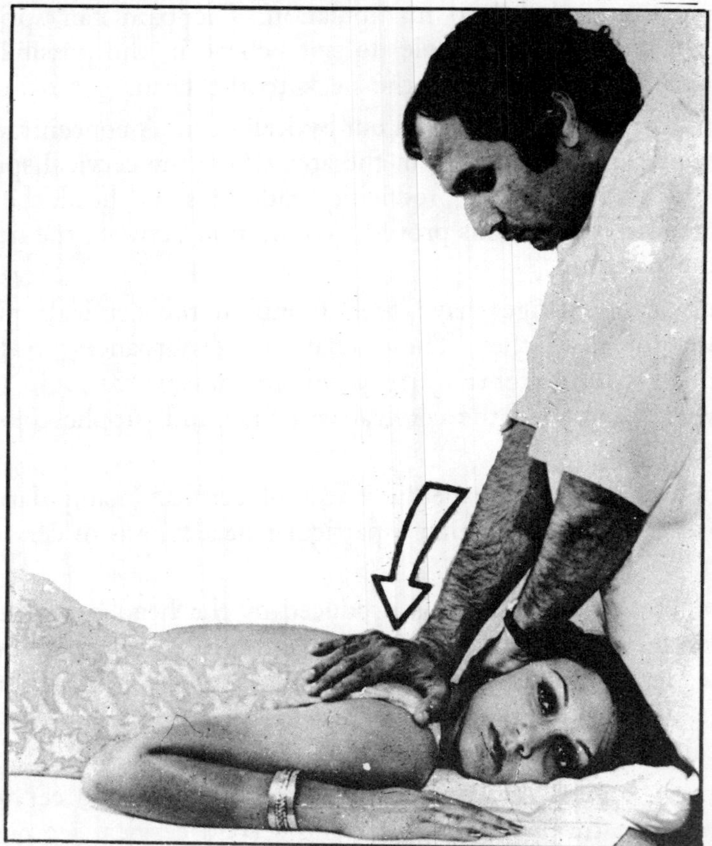

Fig. 20. *Headaches may originate in the neck. Manipulation of the neck can help in curing them.*

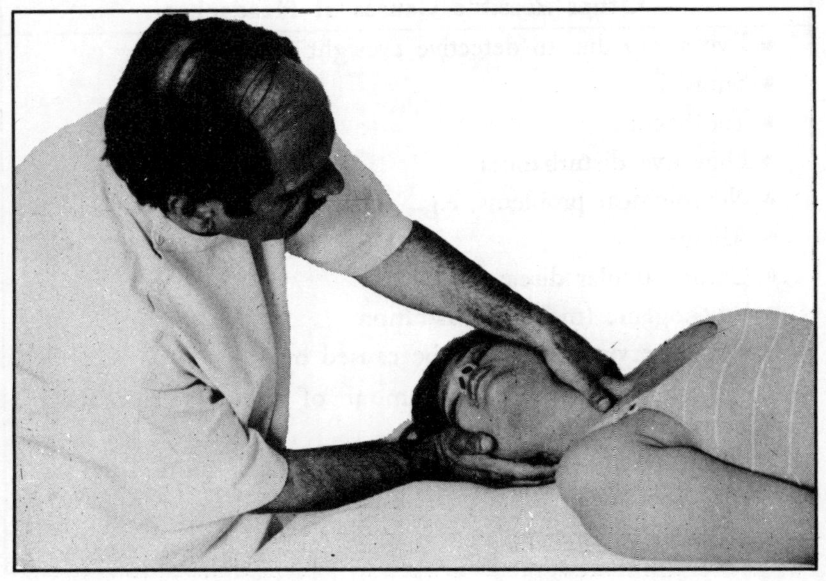

Fig. 21. Treating a migraine.

by, the headache may tend to last longer during the day. It responds well to manipulative treatment.

Dr Bicker's staff is of the opinion that headache is due to stretching or tension in the muscles, vessels or the outermost sheath of the spinal chord. If it is due to these mechanical reasons, the pain starts in the upper neck muscles, and spreads to the upper back and head. Instead of being limited in this area, it spreads to the entire head. It may be associated with stiffness and pain in the upper neck. It occurs off and on. The headache seems to spread from the neck to the head rather than from the head to the neck.

There can be other causes of headaches too. Keeping that in mind, a detailed history of the patient can help in pin-pointing the cause of the headache.

At times differentiation is difficult. But distinction is important, as headaches arising from the neck can most easily and lastingly be relieved. So it is a great pity when the right

Other Possible Causes of Headaches
• Eye strain due to defective eyesight • Sinusitis • Toothache • Digestive disturbances • Neurological problems, e.g., an intra-cranial tumour • Allergy • Cardiovascular diseases • Psychogenic (mental) frustration Upper cervical pain may be caused by: ... An intra-cranial tumour of the posterior fossa (portion) of the skull ... A disease of the upper cervical spine such as tuberculosis ... Malignancy

diagnosis is not made and the right treatment is not administered. An old man is often told that his headache is due to high blood pressure. In fact, it may be completely unconnected and it may be due to upper cervical osteoarthritis. Cervical manipulation can relieve pain on the lateral side of the face. This pain often has rhythmicity and may be associated with a running nose or watering of the eyes. It may radiate to the upper jaw or even the lower jaw. The patient is often referred to a dental surgeon or oral surgeon.

Osteopathic examination may show tenderness over the side of the second and third cervical vertebra on the same side, and if the X-ray picture is clear, manipulation will be successful in many cases and the pain will subside.

Migraine

Headaches occurring at intervals on the right or left side of the head, are associated with nausea and vomiting. There may be a feeling of seeing non-existent objects in front of the eyes before the onset of the headache. Such headaches usually start before the age of 30.

Many such patients respond to manipulation. In some cases migraine may occur at the back of the head. In such cases manipulation will relieve the headache to a considerable degree.

Migraine of Cervical Origin. Spondylosis and osteo-arthritic changes in the cervical spine can cause an inflammatory reaction. This causes a spasm in the vertebral artery and its branches, resulting in a headache with the following characteristics:

1. It is mostly localised in the forehead and may be associated with nausea and severe vomiting. The headache always occurs on the same side. Manipulation elicits a good response.

2. Sometimes the headache is localised at the back of the eyeball and the initial symptoms pertain to visual abnormalities.

Case Histories

❑ A girl, eleven years old, had a severe headache for five days. She underwent laboratory tests of blood, urine, and stool. X-rays were also taken. Every finding was normal and the cause could not be detected. In spite of all possible medication she did not show any improvement. She was thought to be a case fit for a psychiatrist. But her father brought the child to me and narrated the following history: she complained of upper back pain when she went to school with a heavy bag strapped across her shoulders. This pain continued till late evening. She became irritable and would not listen to her parents.

The history of irritability and failure of drugs proved that her ailment was not physical but mental. She was treated manipulatively three times and her headache completely disappeared. She was taught to walk straight instead of going about with a forward stoop. She showed complete recovery.

❑ A 29-year-old lady with three children had been getting headaches off and on since her college days. She also suffered from severe pain in the neck and both shoulders. The headache would occur twice or thrice a month during the day, lasting each time for 10-20 minutes. It would become less during the menstruation cycles. After she got married, the headaches went on increasing in frequency and intensity, and for two years she got headaches every day and had to resort to pain killers. The headaches were accompanied by tension in the neck and were more intense at the back of the head and in the frontal area, in her eyeballs and behind them.

Her condition was diagnosed as migraine. She was given manipulative treatment for her cervical spine and upper dorsal spine. Gradually the headaches started getting less frequent and less intense. She rarely used a pain killer. In 10 weeks the headaches completely subsided.

❑ A 36-year-old engineer employed in the Railways had been suffering from headaches since his school days. They used to occur at fortnightly intervals and later, almost every week. The pain was very severe, starting from the back of the head and then spreading all over the head. He also felt pain in the upper back. His veins became prominent in the temples during the attack, and throbbed. He suffered from nausea and vomiting and would turn away from food or drink. All this would last for twenty-four hours, sometimes even for two to three days. Occasionally, when there was no severe headache, there would be a feeling of general uneasiness. He would prefer to remain in the dark and not be disturbed. He also preferred to lie down till recovery. He was given glasses as his sight was found to be weak, but this did not help. He consulted many doctors and took treatment, but to no avail.

He came to me with his complaint. I examined him thoroughly and found him to have a round upper back. X-rays of the cervical and dorsal spine were taken, but they did not reveal any abnormality; other pathological tests too were all normal.

Manipulative treatment was started. He felt no improvement after the first session. He was called again after a week and manipulative treatment of the cervical and dorsal spine was repeated. He felt some improvement. After a few weeks, his headache became less severe and less frequent. In three months he felt completely recovered, but he continued to come once a month for three months. He has since been advised to come twice a year for maintenance treatment. He has had no attacks ever since.

❑ A young girl aged 21 years suffered from headaches for eight years. At first, she used to have a headache once a month or once a fortnight. During the last three years, the headaches became more frequent and she started having headaches almost every day. The ache was in the entire head, though more severe in the forehead. She did not get nausea or vomiting. Due to the severity of the headaches, she had to discontinue her studies. She was examined by a few doctors but nothing seemed to help her.

She was then referred to me for manipulative treatment. After being treated for three weeks, she felt much better. By the end of six weeks, she was completely cured and the headaches never returned. She has resumed her studies happily.

6
Curing Cervical Spondylosis

Pain in the neck is a common complaint. It is the product of a fast, mechanical life full of tension, lack of exercise and bad posture, use of cushy pillows and a soft bed. It may also be due to an injury. No specific cause can be pin-pointed. Some patients develop a stiff neck due to the incorrect positioning of the head in bed, especially while lying on the tummy with the head turned to one side. Sometimes the pain in the neck lasts for a few days and wears off on its own. But when it persists for a long time, it presents greater problems.

The cervical vertebrae have many peculiarities. They protect the spinal chord which carries practically all the nerves to the whole body. A disease of the cervical spine can have a much wider effect than a similar disturbance in the dorsal or lumbar spine.

The neck has to be mobile and yet it has no support like the ribs in the dorsal spine or the pelvis in the lumbar spine. It has to support the head and a considerable strain is borne by the neck when the arm muscles are put to vigorous use. It carries its own blood supply through the vertebral arteries and veins. These vessels are well protected in transverse processes, but they still experience mechanical problems.

Limitation of movement is one of the main problems. It may occur due to osteoarthritis of the cervical spine, which is called spondylosis. As a person grows old, there is always some generalised wear and tear of bones, including the cervical spine. The most common complaints mentioned are those of pain and stiffness in the neck. These generally occur in the three lowest cervical vertebrae. Patients are not able to turn their necks and look behind. This pain may radiate to the posterior part of the head or upper back between the two shoulder blades and to both shoulders. It is likely that only referred pain is prominent — that is, the patient may not complain of pain in the neck but pain between his shoulder blades only. These patients, especially women, often have swelling in the lower part of the neck. As the swelling subsides there is improvement of mobility and the pain is also reduced or relieved.

In this condition, there is degeneration of the disc between the vertebral bodies. A few osteophytes can be seen at the joint margins in an X-ray. These osteophytes may encroach upon

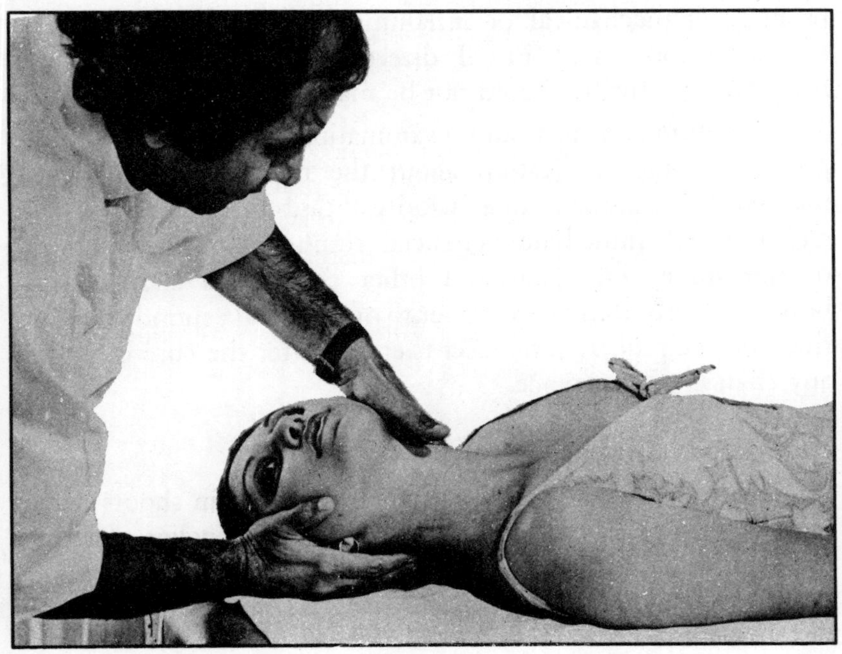

Fig. 22. Treating cervical spondylosis.

the intervertebral foramen (the passages between the vertebrae) and reduce their size. This causes pressure on the cervical nerves. There may be numbness, tingling and a feeling of pins and needles in the hands. There is a tenderness over the muscles of the neck. Occasionally creaking sounds can be heard while moving the neck.

The therapeutic result of manipulation cannot be judged by changes seen in the X-ray. In advanced osteoarthritis excellent results are achieved with the spine recovering its normal range of movement and the pain completely subsiding.

On other occasions, minor changes may take much longer to respond. When osteoarthritis involves facet joints, the results of manipulation are less satisfactory. In such cases manipulation which is too brisk should not be used; the technique must be gentle with a steady progress.

The patient should not be manipulated in an acute phase. A clear cut distinction must be made as to whether the problem is mechanical or inflammatory. In an inflammatory condition movement in all directions is painful. Cases of rheumatoid arthritis should not be manipulated.

A preliminary test and examination of the patient will provide enough indication about the therapeutic success of manipulative treatment. In a majority of cases treatment is possible and induces immediate beneficial results upon the mobility of the spine. The pain and other complaints start getting better. Manipulative treatment of cervical spondylosis is therefore helpful. A few select exercises after the cure diminish any chance of recurrence.

Brachial Neuralgia

Sometimes the arm becomes painful. The pain shoots down one of the arms, accompanied by numbness and a tingling sensation in one or more fingers. This is due to irritation in the nerve roots emerging between the fourth cervical and the second thoracic vertebrae.

There are two factors which cause this pain:

First, pressure of the disc on the nerve root;

Second, inflammation of the nerve sheath or tissue contained in the intervertebral foramen.

The pain may be in the entire upper arm or in a localised area depending upon the site of pressure. It may be a severe pain or a dull pain. It may increase during certain movements of the neck or on laughing. It usually increases when the patient is in bed and is relieved by certain movements, for example, placing one's hand behind one's head.

The patient usually complains of stiffness of the neck and pain between the shoulder blades for years before the disc begins to protrude. When the pain becomes acute, spreading over the upper limb, and the movements get restricted, it is then that the diagnosis of a disc prolapse can be made. A couple of more clinical tests confirm the diagnosis:

1. When the lower part of the neck is involved, movement in the painful side of the neck increases the pain, leading to a numbness in the arm.

2. When traction of the neck provides relief, it confirms the diagnosis.

A symptom frequently accompanying the pain may be in the form of weakness of the neck muscles. Sometimes the pain may be so severe that the patient has to hold his head while sitting. Even while turning his head in bed he may have to support it.

If the pain has started following an injury, the patient may complain of pain several hours after the injury.

The site of pain, numbness, tingling, a feeling of pins and needles, weakening of the neck muscles, decrease in the muscle power and altered reflexes — all depend upon the level of the disc lesion. Clinical and neurological examination can determine the approximate site of the level of disc protrusion.

Treatment

In many cases of brachial neuralgia manipulation is quite effective. When there is acute pain and almost no movement of the neck is possible, manipulation should not be attempted. Prior to manipulation, immobilisation of the neck in a collar, rest and shortwave diathermy may be tried. In some cases where only a little movement is possible, manoeuvres to relax the muscles and gradual mobilisation are helpful. Manipulative manoeuvres should only be attempted when considerable movement in the neck is achieved.

Sometimes manipulation of the upper dorsal spine is also necessary along with cervical manipulation.

In moderate cases manipulation can be started immediately. The treatment must be conducted gently. This is more important in the region of the neck than in any other region.

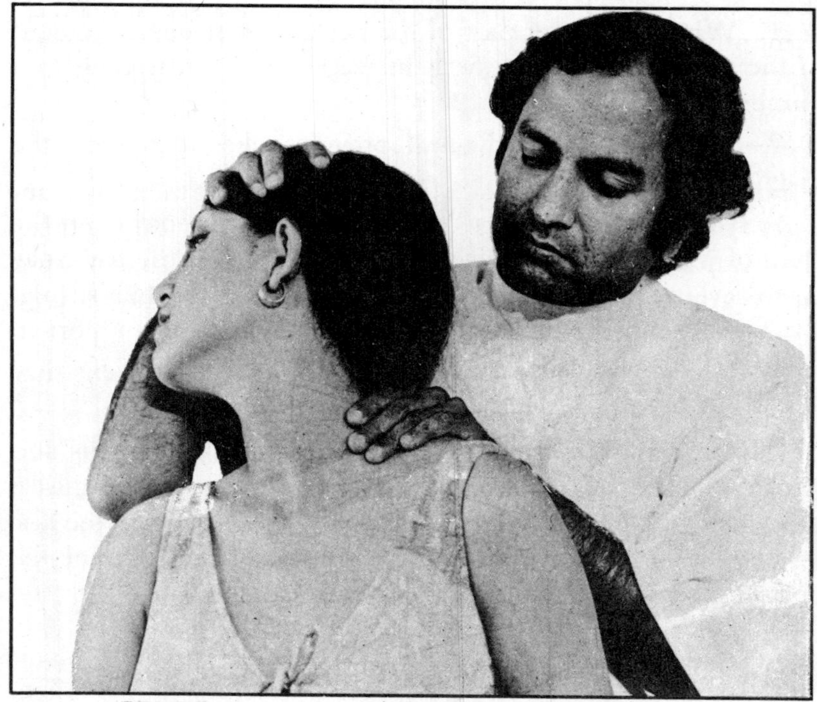

Fig. 23. Neck manipulation in brachial neuralgia.

Selective and gentle treatment is more effective. Thus treatment is given in the following order:

1. Relaxation of the cervical region, shoulders, muscles and upper back.
2. Mobilisation prior to manipulation.

Before manipulation, traction can be utilised, but in cases where traction has failed, manipulation must be given a fair trial.

Following the reduction of disc herniation by manipulation, the patient can use the collar as a protection against strain.

Once the muscle spasm has subsided, the collar can be removed. Other physiotherapy methods may also be used.

Patients should sleep on a hard bed without a pillow. Neck exercises should be started when the pain has completely subsided.

Case Histories

❑ A bankman aged forty-two years suffered for one and a half months from pain in the neck, which radiated to the right arm. He also felt numbness and a tingling sensation in the right arm. He experienced relief by raising his arm but felt more pain when the right arm was hanging down.

He had had a similar attack six years before but then the pain used to radiate to the left arm and subside with cervical traction. The pain, at that time, had lasted for one month. A similar pain had occurred six months ago, which had subsided in fifteen days with the same treatment.

This time the pain was radiating in the right arm and nothing seemed to work in spite of medication and cervical traction.

Manipulative treatment was started. He experienced considerable relief and the numbness and tingling completely subsided. By the third session of the treatment, he was ninety per cent better. In six weeks he had no pain at all and has had no attack since.

❑ A cloth merchant aged forty-eight years complained of neck pain for six months. The pain radiated to the right arm. It was severe for three months. It started without any injury and went on increasing, being present all the time. He felt more pain during the evening after working the whole day. He felt stiffness in the neck when he got up in the morning. Medication and traction of the neck did not help. The X-ray showed no abnormality in the cervical spine. The laboratory tests were all normal.

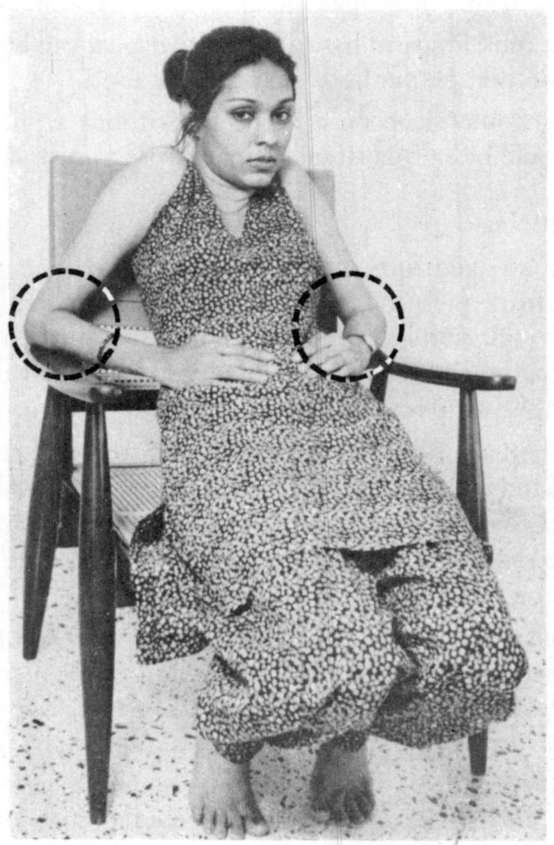

Fig. 24. *One way of relieving pain due to brachial neuralgia: sit on an armchair with the body weight on your elbow and forearm for about 10 minutes before going to bed; this should give you considerable relief and a good sleep.*

He felt a lot of relief for 2-3 days after the first manipulative treatment. The treatment was repeated again after one week and the improvement was remarkable. After four weeks he was free of pain. Now two years have passed and he has had no repetition of pain.

❑ A young housewife from Kanpur, aged twenty-four, had been suffering from pain in the neck for four years. It started without any apparent cause and went on increasing, radiating to both arms, especially when she worked without wearing a collar. She consulted an orthopaedic surgeon and was advised medication and traction, and then given a collar which she used for three years.

When she came to me, an X-ray of her cervical spine was taken again and it showed no change from the previous X-ray. Her laboratory tests were all normal.

Manipulative treatment was started for her cervical and upper dorsal spine. Her pain started getting less from the very first day of treatment. She was advised to use the collar for shorter periods, and that too only when she felt the pain. Within a month, she stopped using the collar. The pain was seventy-five per cent better. She obtained complete relief in two months. A year later I received greetings from her giving me the good news that she no longer suffered from any pain.

7

Curing Postural or Upper Back Pain

A large percentage of patients being treated by general practitioners and being referred to various specialists suffer from back pain. Such patients constitute one-third of the total attendance in the orthopaedic out-patient departments, excluding accident cases. X-rays, electrocardiograms and other investigations are carried out and these patients are then informed that they do not have any serious problem. They are only able to give a vague description of their pain. Unable to find any abnormality in these conditions, the physician treats the problem as a psychological one and often refers them to a psychiatrist.

The pain is mostly in the upper back between the two shoulder blades. It is a postural problem: a wrong way of sitting, standing, or doing home or office work. A majority of sufferers are typists, secretaries and housewives, more commonly females than males. According to our own findings too, such problems occur almost four times more in females than in males. The pain is usually only on one side of the spine. In a few cases it may radiate to the lateral border of the shoulder blade or upwards to the neck. The patient may feel a deep-seated chest pain. Sometimes the pain is excruciating as if somebody is piercing a nail in the back or an abscess is present in the back. At other times it is diffused and a certain heaviness is felt in the back. A few patients describe their pain as a burning sensation or painful tension. Sometimes they point to a specific point on their backs which hurts them the most.

The pain is common in people who use their hands at the level of the chest without providing any support to the elbows. A farm girl doing strenuous work in the field may not get any pain, but when she starts knitting, she may develop a severe pain in the upper back.

Among those who have to do work with a stooping posture or where the posture is not correct, the pain may start — as in the case of a typist sitting and stooping for hours over her typewriter. Housewives who either have a low kitchen platform and have to stoop and work, or sit on the ground stooping and working for hours to cook food, complain that when they roll *chapatis,* they experience pain in the upper back. The pain may be absent while they are engaged in other activities. This pain is common among ladies who use a hand-operated sewing machine or those who iron clothes. Carrying a heavy shopping bag may increase pain. Sometimes the pain may occur at night when the head is in an odd position or when using too high a pillow.

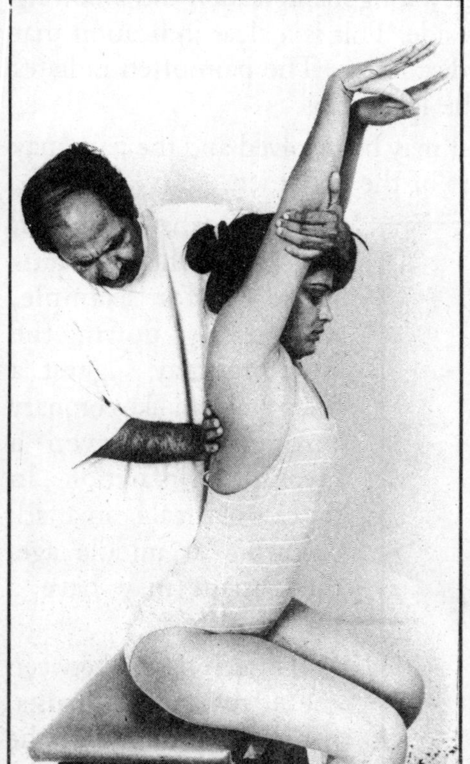

Fig. 25. Examining upper back pain. *The spinal movements are being felt by sensitive fingers.*

Even wearing a heavy overcoat for a long time may bring about pain. The pain is sometimes so severe that the patient cannot carry on with his work.

Pain may also be felt after a sudden twist or turn. It can be severe and excruciating; a deep breath may hurt but coughing may not be painful. This is just the opposite of lumbago (lower back pain) where coughing hurts but deep breathing does not have any effect. A few days of rest may relieve it. While bending the trunk forward, it may recur due to compression on the intervertebral joints. The pain may be felt on one side of the upper back on one occasion, and on the other side on another occasion.

A clicking sound may be felt during manipulation and following this, the pain may change its side. This is a clear indication that thoracic pain is caused by a disc lesion. The pain often radiates to the front at the level of the lower ribs.

Sometimes the whole chest may be involved and the pain may travel down to the upper part of the abdomen.

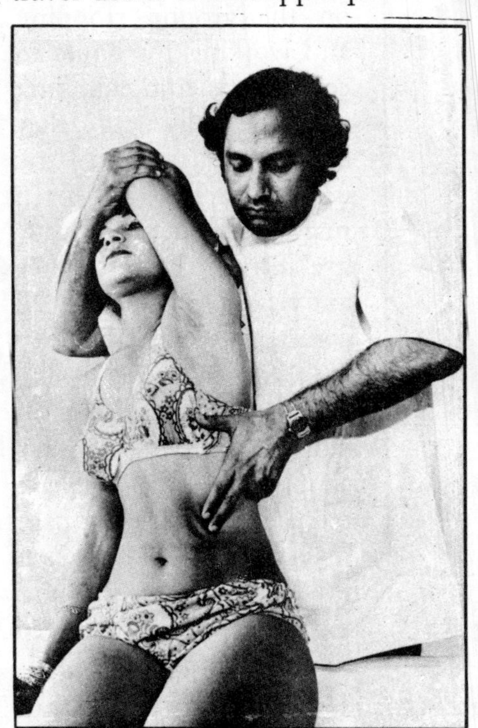

Fig. 26. *Chest pain may be caused by a rib lesion. The treatment lies in the manipulation of the ribs.*

This is when confusion starts. Since the pain starts suddenly, for example, while lying down, the symptom may suggest a heart problem like coronary thrombosis or even a myocardial infarction. In the case of a real heart attack occurring at middle age, the patient may have a similar history.

Differentiation between these two chest pains, namely, a prolapse of the intervertebral disc of the dorsal spine or a real heart attack may be made by asking the patient to take a deep breath. If there is pain during deep breathing, it is most likely that the heart is not involved and the cause of pain is the dorsal spine. An electrocardiogram should also be taken to exclude cardiac involvement. The slipped disc of the dorsal spine is self-curing. It is common among patients like typists, who have to sit for long hours every day. The patient feels comfortable when he wakes up from sleep and for a few hours thereafter; then after sitting for some hours, the pain starts playing up. It goes on increasing as the day wears on. Standing or lying removes the pain in a few minutes. The cause of the pain is the posterior bulging of the disc, which recedes as soon as the forward stoop is no longer there.

When the nerve roots are compressed, the pain may be felt in the lower part of the abdomen or may radiate to the testicles. Sometimes symptoms may appear as in cases of gastritis or cholecystitis, depending on the dorsal involvement. In such cases we should examine the chest and abdomen very thoroughly and any pathological disturbances involving the chest or abdominal organs must be excluded first.

Generally the chest and abdominal symptoms which arise due to pressure on the dorsal nerve root are forgotten while diagnosing different diseases of the chest and abdomen. Most chest or

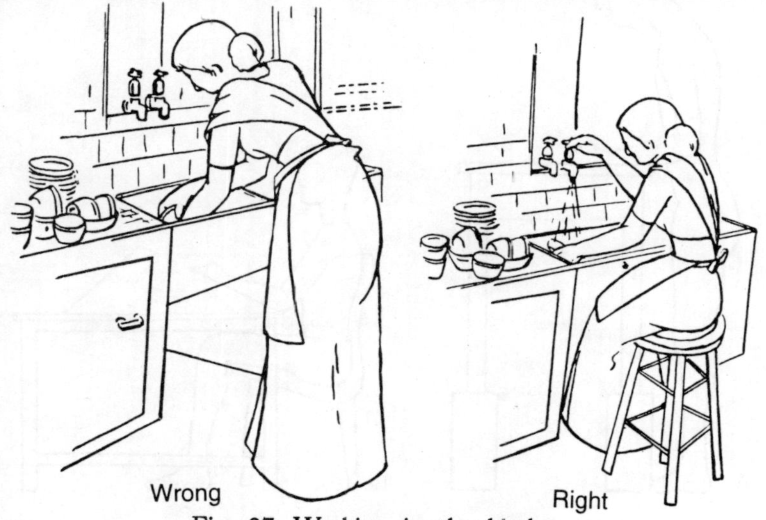

Fig. 27. Working in the kitchen.

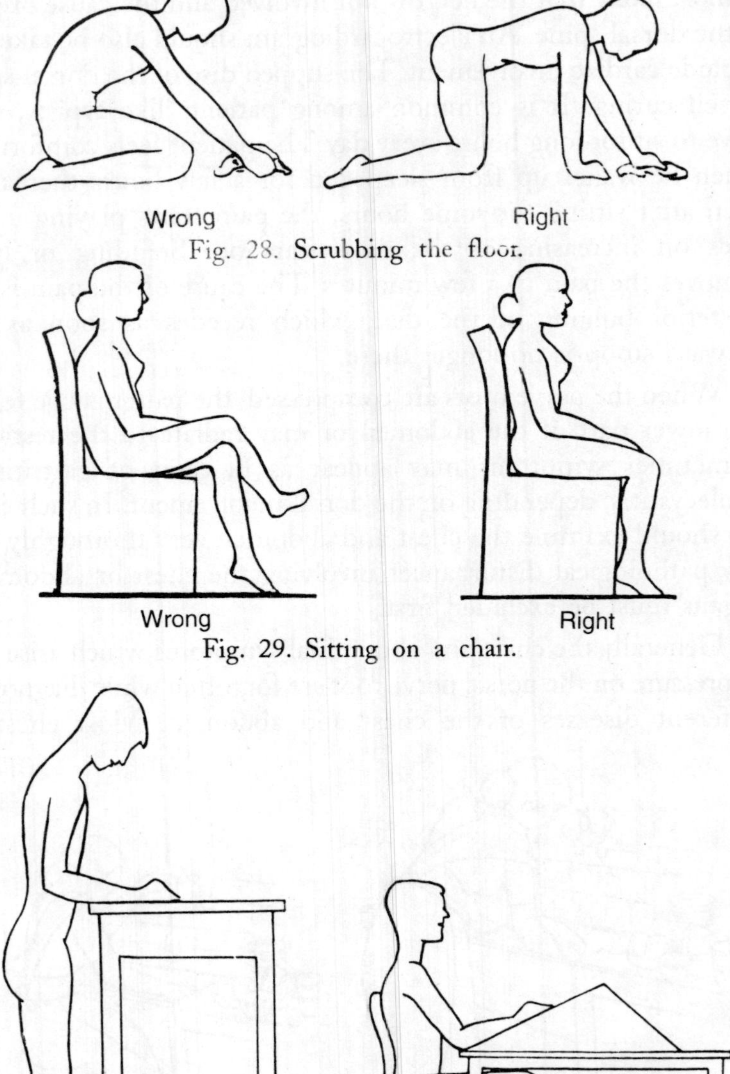

Fig. 28. Scrubbing the floor.

Fig. 29. Sitting on a chair.

Fig. 30. Correct posture. A. *While standing;* B. *Sitting at a slanting desk.*

abdominal pains are due to disease of the local organs, but when the pain is in front of the trunk, and gets aggravated by exertion and bad posture, then you may conclude that it is due to pressure on the dorsal nerve root.

Treatment: Postural Correction

If a straight posture is maintained while working in the office or at home, the pain may not occur. For example, a clerk may raise the height of his table so that he may sit more erect than usual. This can even be done by cutting the legs of the chair to lower its height. A typist may put his or her papers just above the typewriter on an inclined board, or keep them vertically tagged on the wall on a drawing board. Housewives may raise the kitchen platform if it is too low. They may use a *chapati* maker which involves pushing down rather than rolling.

Using a hard bed with no pillow or a very low pillow while sleeping is helpful. Sitting in an ordinary office chair instead of a low sofa is better. One must keep reminding oneself to sit straight as the habit of sitting in a wrong way may be difficult to change. Three exercises are of advantage:

Dand. This is a well-known Indian exercise. The patient rests on his arms and legs. The body is drawn backwards initially, till his hips reach the highest point. This is the starting position. Then the head travels slowly down in the direction of the arms, and after the nose has reached the floor level, the chin and the chest are gradually brought to the same level. Now the upward journey of the head and trunk starts in an arch till the final position of the exercise is reached where the spine is in full extension. This exercise is somewhat difficult. To make it easy, hands should be placed on a higher level than the feet — perhaps on the side of a table or bed. (see Fig. 31). Six repetitions done morning and evening will be very useful.

Shoulder Raise. The patient stands erect with his hands on the side. Both shoulders are raised up and without bringing them down, taken behind as far as possible and then dropped down (see Fig. 32).

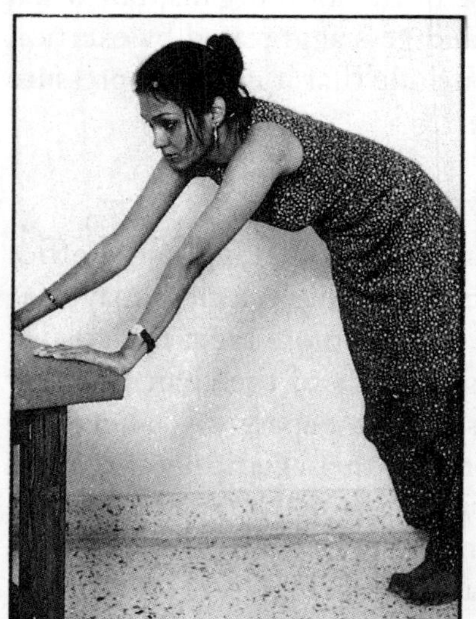

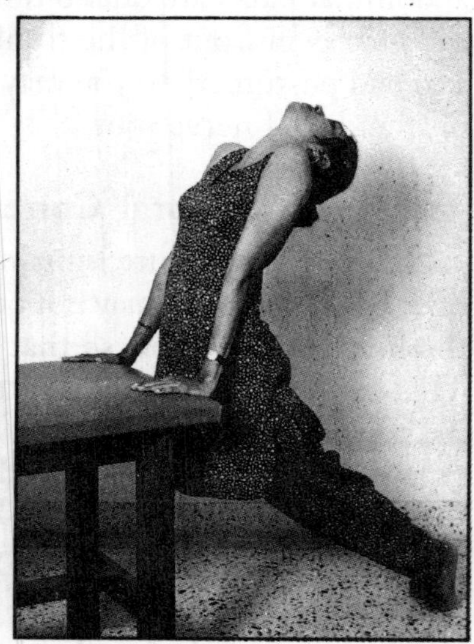

Fig. 31. *Dand (Push-Ups).*

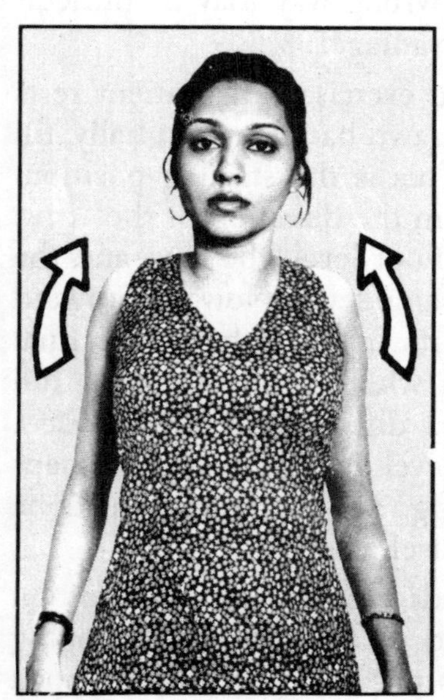

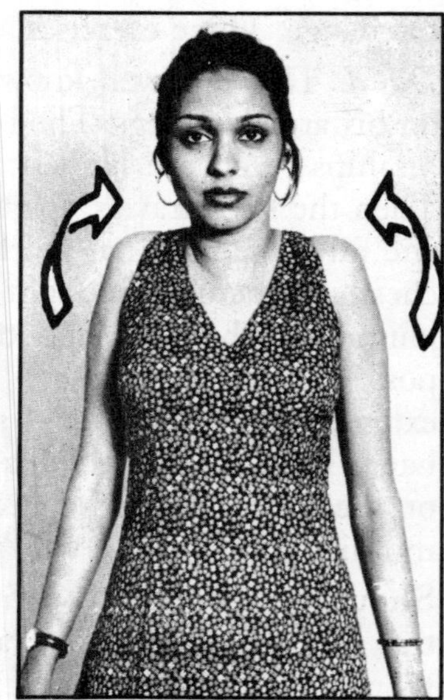

This exercise can be done twelve times in the morning and evening. This also helps to alleviate upper back pain.

Swimming. Swimming helps patients with a postural backache problem. Keeping the head out of water keeps the body in a posture of extension. When the body floats, all the compression strain on the body ceases.

Manipulation

Manipulation is attempted in all cases unless contraindicated. In quite a few cases, a tender point can be located 2 cm from the middle of the spine at the level of the fifth or sixth dorsal spine. Pressure over this point reproduces the exact pain which the patient is complaining of. Some years ago Kellagren injected 1 ml of hypertonic saline solution at the above-mentioned tender point. For a few minutes this injection produced the habitual dorsal pain which the patient had been complaining of. He proved that there was an involvement of the dorsal spine in such pain and, therefore, manipulative manoeuvres were justified for its treatment.

The lower cervical spine involvement as a causative factor for upper back pain has already been discussed in earlier chapters.

Manipulation of the lower cervical and dorsal spine should be done in these cases. Manipulation can be done without general anaesthesia. It should be repeated once a week till final recovery takes place.

Case Histories

❑ A 41-year-old woman with a two-year-old child had occasional pain in the upper back and both shoulders for a year. Then for three months it became continuous and severe. She would get severe back pain after ironing clothes or rolling *chapatis.* Along with pain in the upper back, she felt heaviness in the chest. After resting for 1-2 hours, she felt somewhat better. She underwent treatment from her doctors for a few months but this provided no relief. She then came to me and after a clinical examination and investigations, manipulative treatment was started. Her pain subsided gradually and she was able to do all her household work without any discomfort. It took her eight weeks to complete the treatment. She was asked to do the upper back and shoulder-raise exercises.

- A shop-keeper aged thirty-six, had pain in the chest now and then and a persisting heaviness in the same region. After a year, neck pain also started. Though he had suffered no injury, the pain increased and became persistent. He would also get occasional stiffness in the neck and pain in the arms while lifting heavy objects. However at nights he slept well. Treatment by general physicians and medical consultants did not help him. He consulted an orthopaedic surgeon but to no avail. His chest X-rays and electrocardiogram were normal. The X-rays of the cervical spine and dorsal spine were normal. Laboratory tests were also normal. The manipulative treatment of the dorsal and cervical spine was started. He felt better after the first manipulative manoeuvre. His chest pain became less frequent and much less intense, and the pain in the neck did not occur after the second treatment. The chest pain and heaviness completely subsided after eight weeks. He was told to sleep on a hard bed and without a pillow. He was also told to do exercises.
- An engineer, aged thirty-three, employed with a large company, used to get pain in the lower ribs and chest off and on. This became more prominent when he had to do any job bending for a long time. This pain persisted for two to three days. When he lay flat in bed, the pain subsided slowly. The pain was incapacitating and allowed him no exertion. He would also get pain in the upper back and lower back occasionally. The chest pain followed the low back pain and with this pain he became bed-ridden for fifteen days. X-rays of the chest and electrocardiograms were taken on several occasions but they were all normal. Laboratory tests too did not reveal any significant abnormality.

Manipulation was done on his dorsal spine. The pain subsided in six weeks' time. He could now bend and work for hours without any pain at all. He was also told to do exercises for his back for five minutes every day, and use a hard bed and a low pillow.

- An engineer, aged twenty-nine, met with a car accident while in the US. He started getting pain in the upper back following this accident. The X-ray showed that he had a compression fracture of the fifth dorsal vertebra. He was hospitalised for eight days and later flown to India for treatment. Though he became better and improved, a mild pain continued for about a year. His hectic lifestyle also aggravated the pain.

He came to me with the above complaint. His X-ray showed an old fracture of the dorsal spine. Manipulative treatment was given to him for the cervical and dorsal spine. He improved and there was no pain at all within six weeks. He was taught exercises and advised to be careful about his posture as he was in the habit of sitting and walking with a forward stoop.

8
Curing Low Back Pain, Lumbago and Sciatica

Backache also called lumbago or sciatica, has existed since man learnt to stand erect. Descriptions of the condition occur in ancient literature. Backache is a common complaint among the young and the old. How many people are there who do not suffer from backache during their lifetime? Many suffer from mild, infrequent ache for years before it becomes serious. Many complain of pain after pushing a heavy almirah or lifting something heavy even when they have no injury. Backache may start without any apparent cause. Some ladies complain of pain persisting after a pregnancy. Others complain of pain during their menstrual periods which is severe enough to keep them in bed for 2-3 days and force them to take analgesics.

Human diseases assume importance when they cause death and disability. Lumbago and sciatica do not kill a man, but they are prevalent and cause much suffering.

In Sweden, members of the National Health Scheme report their illness by telephone in order to receive compensation from the Central Bureau. So statistics there are readily available. Back pain has been reported among fifty-three per cent of workers doing light jobs and sixty-four per cent of those doing heavy work. Low back pain is prevalent in the younger age group too. The mean age of the onset of pain is thirty-five years. Among those complaining of low back pain, thirty-five per cent are likely to develop sciatica and ninety per cent will have future reccurrences. Fifty per cent of those suffering from low back pain also complain of pain in the neck, but on an average, they experienced it six years after their low back pain had started. Twenty per cent of them have pain in the thoracic spine.

A clinical and radiological survey of the British town of Leigh revealed that among males between the ages of fifty and sixty-four, eighty-three per cent showed evidence of significant lumbar disc degeneration.

Low back pain can be experienced as follows:

1. Discomfort in the lower back.

2. Severe pain localised in the lower back. This may occur suddenly and is called acute lumbago. When it comes gradually and persists for a long time, it is called chronic lumbago.

3. Pain radiating from the lower back to the posterior part of the thigh and calf. It may radiate only up to the buttocks, or it may radiate to the anterior aspect of the thigh when the higher lumbar area is involved. This is called sciatica.

It is quite spectacular to see a patient who is bent over as a result of pain, recover instantaneously following manipulation. These manoeuvres appear to be very simple; only the click sound is often heard during manipulation. It is generally considered that lumbago occurring in young people is the most obvious symptom for manipulation. However such cases sometimes recover after simple bedrest. But more severe cases of sciatica, persisting for years, and with no obvious sign of subsiding, improve with manipulation.

Let us examine the case of a patient with a typical history of acute lumbago. The patient probably felt pain and heard a clicking sound while lifting a heavy object from the ground. (This may also happen while pushing a heavy object like an almirah.) The pain became severe and the patient was unable to move. A few days later, the pain became less severe, but radiated to the buttocks, the back of the thigh, and the calf and foot. Tingling and numbness were felt in the leg. There was severe pain while sneezing or coughing.

A patient with these symptoms and acute back pain adopts a peculiar posture. Muscles in the lower part of the back look prominent as they are contracted in an effort to immobilise the painful spine. The patient tries to assume a posture of maximum comfort. He may develop a lateral curve. The curve may also get obliterated and become straight. The patient finds it difficult to bend forward or backward. Lateral bending is not so painful. He is not able to raise the painful leg high while lying on his back. A careful examination may reveal that there is wasting of the muscles. The corresponding tendonous jerks are impaired or absent.

In a few cases the pain can start without any history of injury, and the onset may be gradual. It may be confined to the back only and not travel to the legs. Sometimes a patient does not feel any pain in the lower back. He may feel it only in the legs and calf muscles. In cases where a higher lumbar disc is involved, the pain radiates to the groin or to the front of the thigh.

Patients with a prominent belly have increased anterior convexity of the lumbar spine. They have more prominent buttocks and a belly. They feel pain while standing and while bending backwards, and experience relief when they sit or bend forward, or when they lie on one side with the knee and hip bent upwards. In such cases more weight is carried by the posterior arches than by the vertebral body and disc. These arches are not meant to bear weight, hence wear and tear in the facet joints starts. This may affect the intervertebral foramen, and put consequent pressure upon the nerves.

Treatment

It is most important to ascertain that the pain is of vertebral origin. Pain due to infection, inflammation, tuberculosis, tumour of the spine, osteomyelitis, cancer or other diseases should be excluded.

A sudden dramatic pain is most likely due to a derangement of the spine. Pain which increases relentlessly without any intermission suggests that it may be due to inflammation or malignancy. In such cases, an X-ray has to be done to check out the condition of the spine and the disc. However if there is an acute prolapse, the X-ray may not show any abnormality, but may show the extent of osteoarthritis as being extensive or mild. It may be remembered that there are many patients with the same radiological changes who do not experience pain, and they continue to show the same changes even after they obtain complete relief.

An injury or strain may indicate the time when the annulus fibrosus of the disc was torn. The nucleus pulposus will bulge from this torn annulus. As the nucleus pulposus is gelatinous, there is a time gap between the injury and the advent of acute pain. If this bulging material lies behind the posterior longitudinal ligament, the patient suffers from acute lumbago; if the nucleus pulposus herniates through the weakened ligament, it impinges on the nerves and there is radiation of pain in the lower limb.

Acute lumbago may also be due to other mechanical disorders of the spine: the sudden nipping of the synovial membrane in one of the facet joints; or subluxation due to constant ligamentous strain, bad posture, disc degeneration or osteoarthritis.

There is great controversy among doctors and orthopaedic surgeons regarding the treatment of lumbago. Some may not allow their patients to be manipulated at all, while others may manipulate each and every case under general anaesthesia. At a meeting of the World Orthopaedic Association, a panel of seven experts under the chairmanship of Professor Mc Farland discussed the problem: even though thirty-three per cent of all orthopaedic outpatients complained of low back pain, the panel had no unanimous suggestions for coping with such a vast number.

Treatment of low back pain is controversial. There is no other condition where treatment varies so much from doctor to doctor. Moreover, treatment depends more on the severity of the symptoms rather than on the severity of the lesion. The arbiter of the result is the patient himself, and different patients have varying sensitivities towards pain.

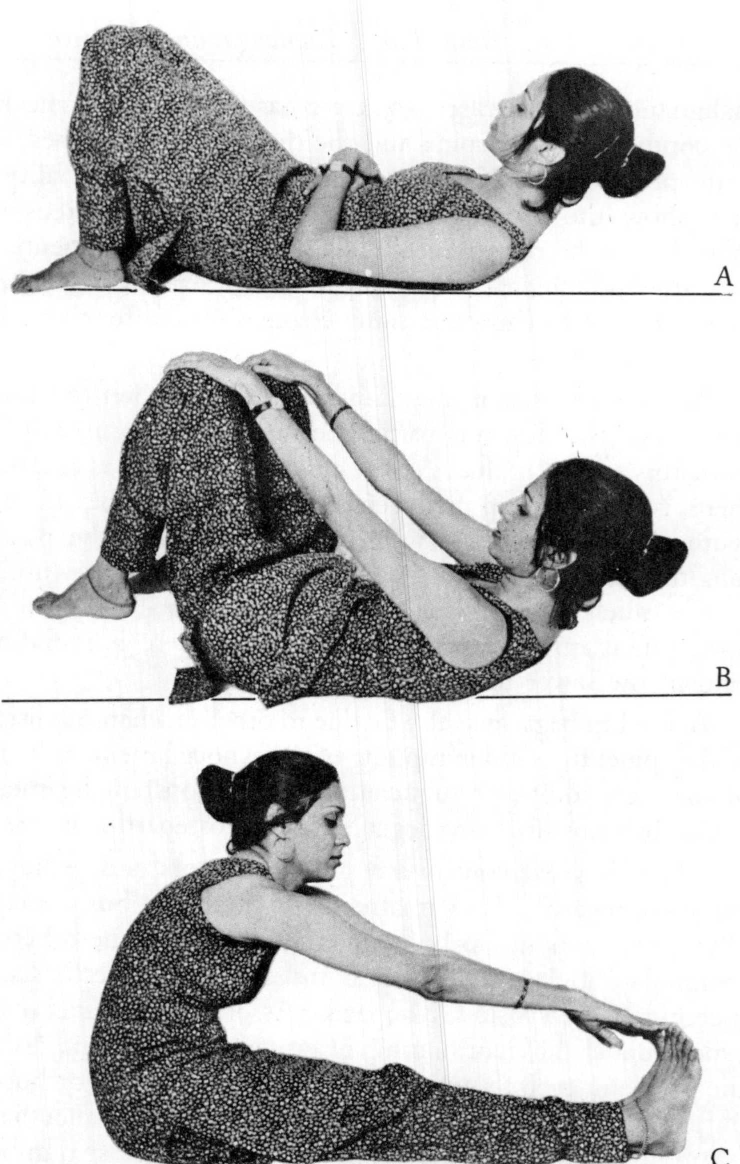

Fig. 33. Exercises for low back pain. A. *Lie on your back with knees bent and feet flat on the floor. Place hands on the abdomen. Raise your head and upper part of your back while contracting the abdominal muscles;* B. *Lie on the back, separate legs, separate knees and hips, and draw knees up towards the underarms by clasping them with hands;* C. *Sit on the floor with legs outstretched. Touch your toes without bending knees. When able to touch your toes, stretch beyond toes.*

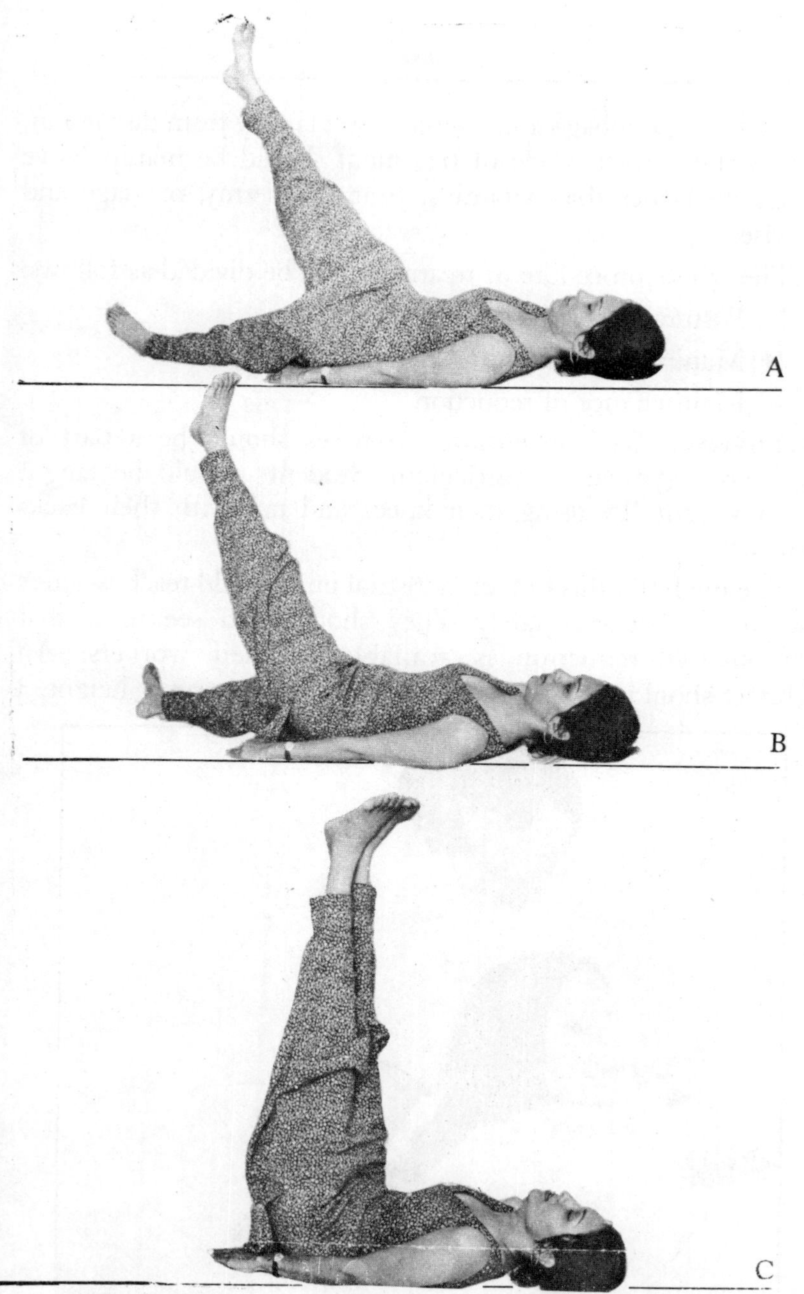

Fig. 34. Exercises for low back pain. *Lie flat on your back without bending the knees, hands flat on your sides.* A. *Lift one leg straight up, bending at the hip;* B. *Then the other;* C. *Then both together. Do these exercises three times at a stretch and gradually increase to 12 times. Do them twice a day.*

Backache, lumbago and sciatica result largely from disc lesion, and so the correct mode of treatment should be manipulative reduction, rather than vitamins, heat, diathermy, massage and exercise.

The whole procedure of treatment can be divided as follows:

1. Postural prophylaxis
2. Manipulative reduction
3. Maintenance of reduction

Prophylaxis. Back extension exercises should be a part of the school gymnastics curriculum. Students should be taught to lift weights by using their knees and not with their backs arched.

The medical officer in an industrial unit should teach workers how to lift weights safely. They should also see to it that manipulative reduction is available to their workers. An architect should see that the sink is placed at a proper height, a

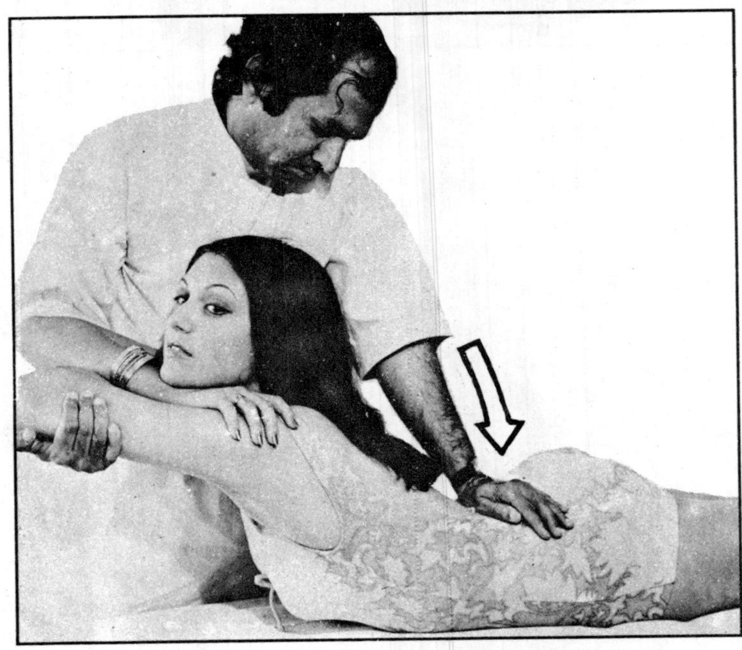

Fig. 35. Treatment of low back pain.

little higher than customary. The car seat too should be designed in a way that the right posture is maintained.

Patients must be instructed not to do toe-touching exercises. It is much better to do extension exercises so as to keep the muscles strong. If a patient is engaged in heavy work and has had several relapses, the employer must be asked to give him a lighter job.

Manipulation

If the pain is of recent origin and started after bending down or lifting a weight or pushing an almirah, why should it not be cured in an equally short time? The treatment of a slipped disc by manipulative treatment is logical and ethical. Treatment should be by manipulative reduction. But before manipulation, a definite diagnosis should be made and all contraindications for manipulation excluded through the patient's history, clinical examination, X-ray and laboratory tests. If there is any doubt about the diagnosis, it is better to postpone manipulative treatment.

Manipulation should not be done if a patient has acute pain and is not able to move in bed. A few days' bedrest and formentation should follow manipulation. Different variations of manipulative procedure are adopted to suit each individual case. In the case of sciatica, a mechanical irritation of the nerve by the disc after intermittent pressure, produces inflammation and swelling of the nerve. This leads to pain and an abnormal sensitivity in the area distributed by the nerve. Adhesions around the nerve roots are formed and often remain even after the inflammation has completely subsided; then the pain is felt only when the nerve is stretched.

The secondary effect of nerve root irritation or compression arises when the patient tries to escape pain by adopting a position of comfort. In this process different curvatures in the spine, called scoliosis, may occur. If there is no inflammation, the patient is able to adopt a pain-free position. If the nerves are inflamed and swollen, the pain increases during the night. Once mechanical

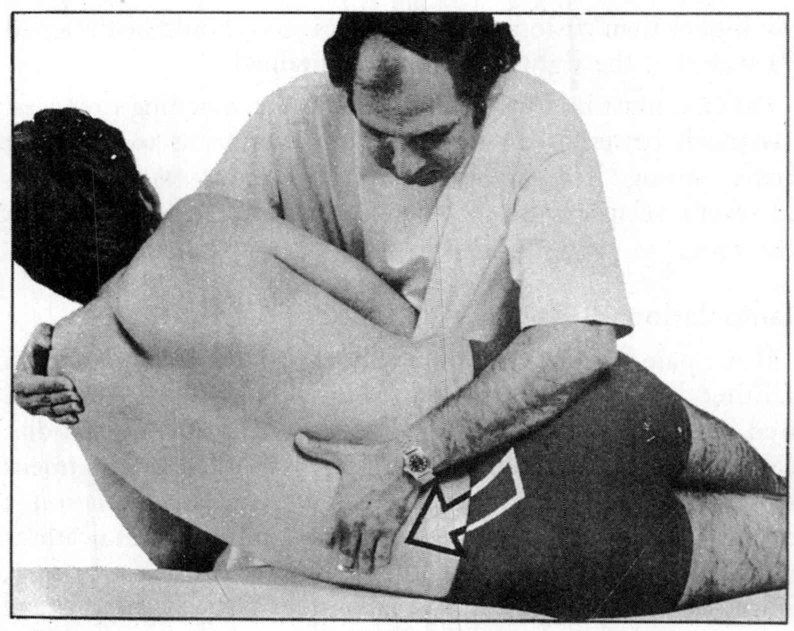

Fig. 36. Treatment of lumbar pain.

irritation leads to inflammatory change, the rate of recovery is slow and the pain is prolonged.

The treatment in such cases is as follows:

1. Removal of pressure from the nerve through manipulation
2. Avoidance of further irritation
3. Treatment of residual muscle weakness, if any
4. Precaution against recurrence

Here is a very recent report which should be used as a guide before deciding whether we should resort to surgical interference in disc cases or not.

The Karolinska Institute, USA, made a study of 583 patients after their first attack of sciatica. Surgery was performed on twenty-eight per cent of them. A close watch was kept on the groups of both operative and non-operative patients for seven years. The study showed that an acute attack of sciatica ran a relatively similar brief course in most cases, regardless of whether the treatment had been conservative or surgical.

There is a noteworthy reduction in the number of disc operations being performed the world over. This is due to the poor results obtained and complications following such operations.

A neurological deficit including muscle and motor weakness, is not a compelling factor for surgical interference. Uncontrolled urine and bowel movement which occurs in a small number of cases, however, does call for surgical interference.

Surgery should not be done if the pain is severe. It is much better to wait. It should only be considered in cases where manipulative manoeuvres have been tried and failed. When the pain is severe, a pillow can be put under the knee. A few patients may find a sitting position more comfortable.

Complete bedrest and traction should be given and continued till the pain is reduced. But if the pain persists after two weeks of bedrest, manipulative reduction to shift the pressure upon the nerve can be attempted.

If there is a deformity in the spine, sustained traction is often effective at the acute stage. Bedrest and traction should be continued till the pain subsides.

Patients may need the support of a corset, but it should not be used for more than 3-4 weeks, otherwise, the lower back muscles become weak, and strengthening them later on becomes a problem.

When the pain has subsided, exercises should be started. If a particular exercise causes pain, it should be avoided. The aim should be to increase muscle strength. A soft bed and low chairs should also be avoided.

Posture

The patient should be taught how to use his knee joints so as to avoid over-bending. He should be made to sit and rise again with the object being lifted.

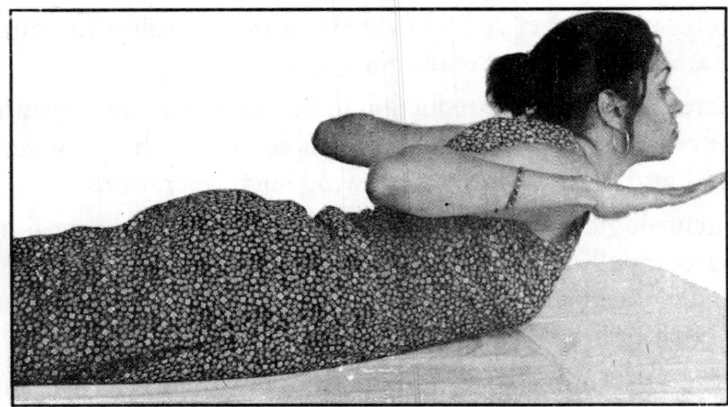

Fig. 37. Exercise for low back pain.

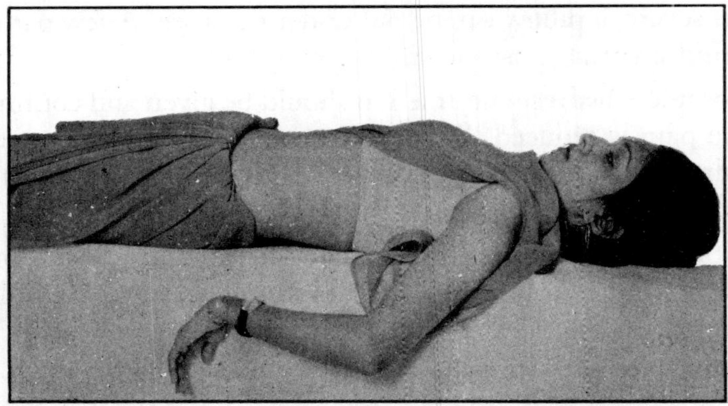

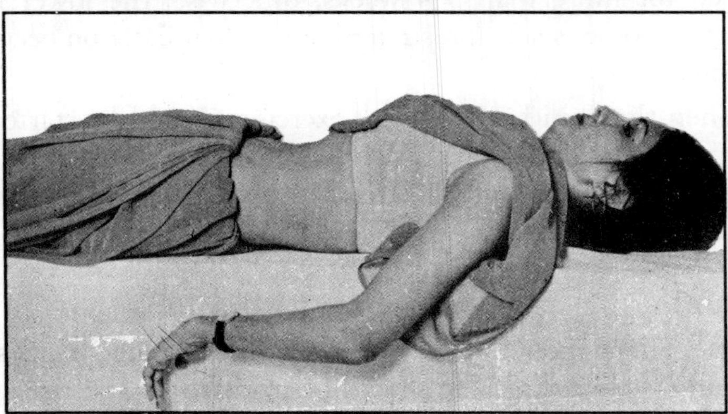

Fig. 38. Correction of lumbar lordosis.

When turning, the patient should avoid twisting his body. It is much better to change the position of the feet instead and change direction.

Lumbar and abdominal exercises must be demonstrated. It is better to do one simple exercise than a set of exercises.

Exercises

1. Lie on your tummy. Place your hands flat on the ground in front with shoulders back, and lift your shoulders and head up as far as you can. Hold the position for 10 seconds, return to rest for 5 seconds, then repeat the exercise again. Repeat it 20 times morning and evening. If it hurts, do it a less number of times and increase the number by one every day (see Fig. 37).

2. If the tummy is big, it also pulls forward the lumbar spine, causing a constant strain. Reduce your tummy by lying on your back. Keep your arms on your side; lift your leg upto about 45° to 70°, or even to 90°, and bring it down again. Repeat this 20 times. Do it morning and evening (see Fig. 34).

3. Correction of lordosis is important. The patient should lie on his back. He should pull in his abdomen and hold his buttocks close together to push his lower back against the floor, and then relax and start it over again. This may be done for 2-3 minutes at a time and 3-4 times a day. It must be done on the floor or on a wooden plank with a rug over it. It should not be done on a mattress (see Fig. 38).

Case Histories

- During a series of test matches played between India and the MCC, the opening batsman was found to be suffering from back pain on the first day of the first test match. As a result, he could not play in the match. He thought that the pain was due to sleeping in an air-conditioned room. His pain persisted in spite of the best possible treatment. All possible investigations were done and X-rays taken. Finally he was diagnosed as having a slipped disc of the lumbar spine, and advised complete bedrest for three weeks. When he did not improve, his bedrest was extended for a further three weeks. Later he was referred to the physiotherapy department for shortwave diathermy and traction. He was also given a belt to wear and asked to do exercises which he did very vigorously since he was keen that his career should not be ruined. He was asked to undergo a disc operation. He refused this fearing that though the operation might rid him of the pain, he would never return to the cricket grounds as he would never be able to reach the required efficiency needed for a world-class batsman.

He started treatment with an expert masseur who gave him a massage every day for half an hour, for six weeks. This too did not help much. He still had pain while walking, and the pain would start after sitting for a while in a chair.

Then he came to me for osteopathic treatment. I started him on manipulative treatment of the lumbar spine. He was recalled after one week. His anxiety was great as the time for the team selection at Madras for the Australian tour was approaching fast.

He began showing improvement within six weeks; started playing inter-club matches every Sunday and doing his Keep-Fit exercises. At the end of eight weeks, he was ready to leave for Madras. His performance was good. There was no end to his joy when he scored the highest number of runs in the semi-finals of the Duleep Trophy match.

He was selected for the finals and was grateful to osteopathy, which had put him back on the field.

- For one year a thirty-year-old housewife with a seven-year-old child suffered from low back pain which descended to her right leg. She also experienced pain during her periods. Stiffness of the upper back and neck followed, and lately, she had also started complaining of heaviness in the head. She was a keen sportswoman and used to a great deal of cycling. The pain had started after she had pushed a heavy almirah.

She came to me and after being given osteopathic treatment for six weeks, she recovered. Her periods also became free of pain.

- A lady advocate, 28 years old, was bedridden with severe backache. She had no injury preceeding this pain. The pain had started suddenly one day when she got up from bed. Before that she used to get feverish in the evening. The X-rays, ESR and other investigations showed normal results. She did not respond to drug therapy, rest, traction or diathermy. She was also pregnant. Since she was running a temperature, her case was diagnosed as one of tuberculosis. She was advised antitubercular treatment and an abortion. Her family was upset as it was her first pregnancy. A high sacral belt was given to her. This was the time when she came to me.

I examined her. As every investigation and the X-ray were normal, I could not agree with the diagnosis of tuberculosis. I felt that her temperature was due to severe pain and decided on manipulative treatment for her spine. She responded well. The next time she came to me, she did so without a stretcher. She could walk from the portico to my consulting room. By the end of the third treatment she was a lot better and definitely hopeful. At the end of six weeks, she was back to work. Two more sessions of treatment at fortnightly intervals included back extension exercises.

No abortion was done, and she delivered a normal healthy baby. It was a painless delivery.

- A man aged 49 complained of low back pain which radiated to the right leg. It began when he tried to lift something heavy from the ground. He took medication, rest and traction, but all these did not help. He took recourse to auto-urine therapy for ten days but this did not seem to help either. He went to Poona and got himself thoroughly examined. An X-ray was taken and his lumbar spine was manipulated three times under general anaesthesia, but this too did not help. Ultimately he was brought to me. He could not even sit. After examination I gave him manipulative treatment. He felt much better after the first session. The third time he came for treatment he was able to travel by train and bus. By his sixth visit, he was able to resume his insurance work. He recovered completely after two months.

❑ A well-built mechanic, 41 years old, complained of pain in the calf muscles for fifteen years. He had pain in the upper back and both shoulders for eight years. But there was no injury. The pain was present all the time, sometimes a little less, sometimes more. He was better if he rested at home; otherwise, it would start in the morning and increase by evening. There was no numbness or tingling in the legs. He had difficulty even walking short distances. After having tried several types of treatment and undergone other investigations, manipulative treatment was finally started.

He felt much better following the first treatment. He showed improvement, and by the end of six weeks he had no pain at all. He was advised to sleep on a hard bed and keep on doing exercises for his back.

9
Curing Shoulder Pain

'Doctor, I don't know what has happened to my shoulders. They ache a lot and the ache is gradually increasing. I cannot move them properly. It is becoming impossible for me to put on my clothes myself. Even combing has to be done by somebody else. The pain persists during the day, but at night it becomes worse. If somebody presses my shoulder joint, I get an excruciating pain. I have had all kinds of treatment but nothing seems to be helping me. Can you do something?'

The above symptoms seemed to point towards a frozen shoulder. This condition can be diagnosed easily. The shoulder joint is frozen and its mobility reduced. Before we go further let us examine what our shoulder joints are and what they do.

A shoulder joint is a ball and a socket joint. The head of the upper arm bone (humerus) and a shallow cup-like structure of the shoulder blade (scapula) make up this joint. The head is much bigger than the socket and only a part of the head can fit into the socket called the glenoid cavity. The socket is deepened by a fibro-cartilagenous rim. Due to this arrangement, the shoulder has a better range of movement than any other joint in the body. But it is a weak joint and depends on the surrounding muscles for its strength.

The joint is covered by a sac-like structure, a fibrous capsule. This capsule is lax and the bones can be separated from each other for a distance upto half an inch. This can provide a further range of movement. The inferior part of the capsule is the weakest part. The movement at the shoulder joint is further increased by the movement of the shoulder blade itself. When the arm is raised upto 120°, movement takes place at the shoulder joint and a further 60° is obtained by rotation of the shoulder blade. The acromio-clavicular joint at the lateral end of the collar bone (clavicle) and sterno-clavicular joint at the medial end of the collar bone also participate in shoulder movements.

In the case of a frozen shoulder, the capsule is thickened and retracted. This can be clearly demonstrated by arthography (taking an X-ray after injecting a radio-opaque dye inside the joint).

Why a frozen shoulder occurs is not known. There is a limitation of movement in all directions. It generally occurs between the ages of forty to sixty. After sixty, it is rare. The usual course of the disease is as follows:

It starts with an ache in the shoulder when the arm is moved. There is pain when the arm is kept still. After one month the pain is more severe and spreads down to the elbow. It is worse at night and increases further if the patient lies on the same side. Restriction of movement starts becoming obvious. After 2-3 months severe pain occurs at the slightest movement. The patient cannot raise his hand more than thirty to forty degrees. The rotative movement of the arm is also limited. After 4 months no further diminution takes place in the movement. The pain is at its worst at the end of 4 months. After 5 months it begins to reduce gradually. After 6 months there is no constant pain. Pain is felt only when the arm is moved. The patient is now able to lie on the painful side. After 7 months there is pain only in the upper part of the shoulder. After 8 months the range of movement begins to become wider. After one year the patient is almost well.

It has been noted that the pain and restriction of movement decrease during the first four months. During the next four months the pain decreases but the limitation of movement persists. In the last 4 months the range of movement returns. If exercises are done, the full range of movement is sure to return, and if no exercises are done, some amount of permanent limitation will persist at the shoulder joint.

In the severe variety, pain may go on increasing upto nine months. Wasting and thinning of muscles also start and complete recovery may take upto two years.

Treatment

Some doctors advise forced mobilisation under general anaesthesia. Though some very good results have been achieved by this process, some grave setbacks also occur. This treatment is therefore not advisable because during this act a tear in the lower part of the capsule can occur. This has been seen by arthography taken before and after the treatment. We believe that skill and experience play a dominant role in achieving good results. It is very important to know when to stop and how to grade these manoeuvres. This is practically impossible when the manipulation

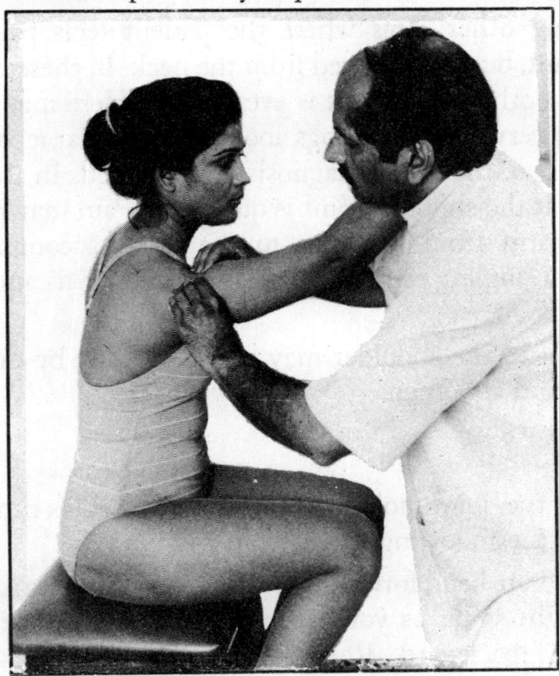

Fig. 39. Stretching in the case of a frozen shoulder.

is done under anaesthesia, because the results are only known the next day or when the patient wakes up. For such cases we recommend a gradual stretching of the shoulder without anaesthesia. However this is not as simple as it sounds. If there is too much stretching, it provokes pain and if there is too little, it does not produce any results. Stretching has to be done with great care. The patient feels great discomfort when the arm reaches the restricted range; it should then be coaxed a little further without increasing the pain or producing a muscle spasm. The shoulder should be moved in this final increased range for five to seven minutes twice a week. The patient should also be taught certain exercises which should be done twice a day at home. This treatment, in my experience, reduces the recovery period to two to three months. Sometimes cervical and upper dorsal manipulation along with mobilisation is helpful.

This treatment can also be given in the case of a frozen shoulder after an accident.

There are other cases where the patient feels pain in the shoulder joint, but it is radiated from the neck. In these cases, 'the shoulder is nothing, the neck is everything!' Here manipulation of the lower cervical spine brings about a spectacular recovery, and when this is so, the above diagnosis is confirmed. In these cases movement at the shoulder joint is quite free. Pain may radiate in the whole arm from the base to the neck, accompanied by numbness, a tingling sensation and a feeling of pins and needles in the hands.

The pain in the shoulder may also be caused by diseases of the thorax and abdomen.

Exercises

Keeping the joint mobile is very important. This can be done at home in the following way:

1. Stand up, bend forward, leave your arm hanging loose, take it to the right as far as you can, then to the left. Then take it forward and backward. Rotate the arm clockwise and anti-clockwise. Repeat this twenty times. (Fig. 40, A & B).

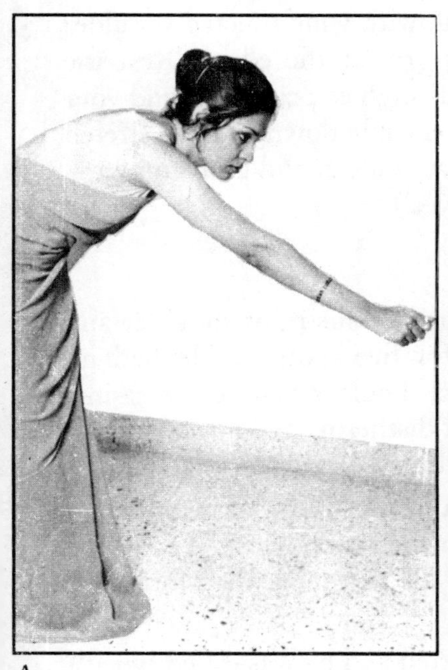

A

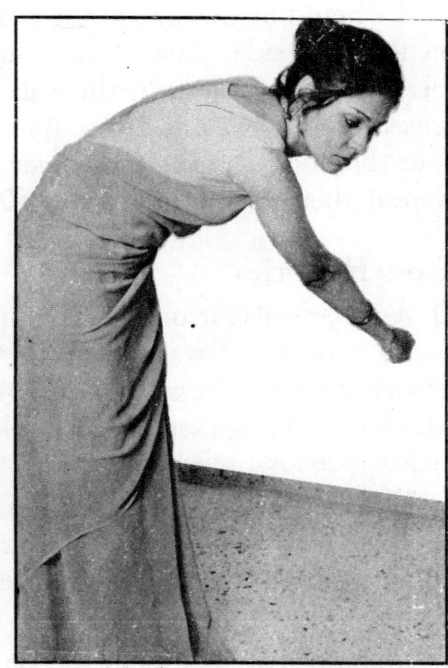

B

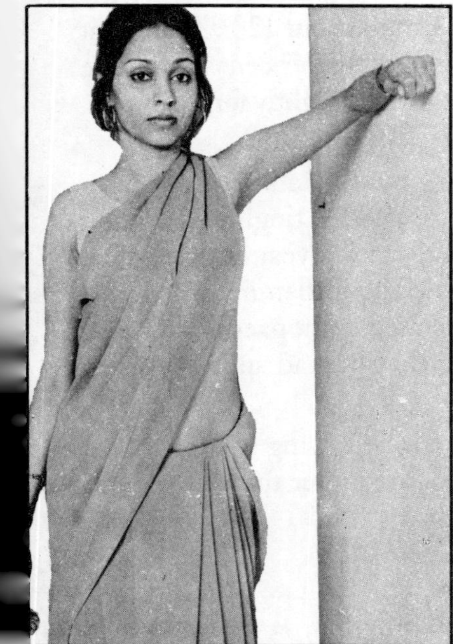

C

Fig. 40. Exercises for a frozen shoulder. A. *Take the arm forward and backward;* B. *Take the arm from left to right;* C. *Stretch your arm up.*

2. Stand by the side of the wall, with your affected shoulder on the wall side. Now bend your arm at the elbow. Rest the forearm on a platform by the wall as high as possible. Bend your knees and slowly come down. As you come down you will stretch your shoulder up. Go down as far as you can and then come up. Repeat this twenty times (Fig. 40, C).

Case Histories

❑ A fifty-five-year old man had pain in his right shoulder and his movement was restricted for five months. He had no history of injury. The pain in the right shoulder went on increasing. Along with doing exercises, he took diathermy and intra-articular hydro-cortisone injections, but nothing helped.

He came to me with this complaint. The X-ray of his shoulder joint was clear: the cervical spine showed spondylosis. The blood sugar was high. He could not raise his arm more than forty-five degrees.

Manipulative treatment was started and he was called twice a week. He was taught a few exercises to be done at home. By the end of three weeks, he could raise his arm to about 120°. Treatment continued for two months and he was ninety per cent better. He was advised to continue exercises and come fortnightly for treatment. Two months later he was completely free of pain.

❑ A thirty-eight-year old man, thinly built, had a severe pain in the left shoulder radiating to the arm, with a tingling sensation in the left hand. He had had a similar attack a year before which had cleared in two months. He took anti-inflammatory drugs which gave him little relief. He consulted orthopaedic surgeons and an X-ray was taken, confirming that he had spondylosis of the cervical spine.

Manipulative treatment was started. Following the treatment he had no pain for four days. He was cured after the third round of manipulative treatment.

10
Curing Elbow Pain

A patient may complain that he cannot pour a cup of tea for himself. He experiences difficulty in closing his fist tightly, or while grabbing and lifting heavy things from the ground with his hands. He has pain on the lateral aspect of the elbow at a prominent point called the lateral condyl of the humerus or arm bone. The pain travels along the back of the forearm and may go as far as the wrist or the back of the hand as far as the ring finger of the hand. It may be severe enough to go to the external aspect of the arm up to the shoulder, but this is less common. Sometimes, there is a constant ache, which gets worse at night, disturbing the sleep. The patient may wake up with stiffness of the elbow.

Tennis Elbow

Pain at the elbow joint is commonly seen among tennis players. That is why this condition is commonly called *tennis elbow*. Those who do not play tennis may also suffer from elbow pain.

The pain starts due to a strain where the wrist has to be extended again and again as is done while playing tennis or while using the hammer. The patient does not feel any pain even after a slight injury to the elbow joint is sustained during these movements. Later on, certain movements at the wrist joint or elbow start hurting and a fortnight later, a tennis player cannot hit backstrokes at all.

It is not the tear of the tendon which causes the pain. The pain is due to the formation of a painful scar which results from multiple injuries. During the game or due to the active use of the elbow and wrist, the healing process which is accelerated by rest and avoidance of movement, remains incomplete. The strain on the extension ligaments is caused during the extension or backward bending at the wrist joint. The pain is peculiar; occasionally it comes on suddenly and the grip of the hand becomes powerless momentarily. The patient may even drop light objects that he is holding on the ground.

Getting a tennis elbow is frequent between the ages of forty to sixty years, the years when cervical spondylosis is also common. A view is often expressed that elbow pain has some relation with the neck. Sometimes this is true. Pain in the elbow joint can arise from the neck without any injury at the elbow. All cases of elbow pain should be examined for a neck lesion too. Generally tenderness can be located at the level of the fifth, sixth and seventh cervical vertebrae. Marked tenderness is noted in the lower part of the neck on the side of the elbow involved. So if the pain in the elbow joint is due to the neck, manipulation of the latter will result in a spectacular recovery. A distinction must be made between elbow pain due to the cervical spine and pain due to a tennis elbow. Sometimes an elbow pain is due to both a cervical lesion and periarthritis of the elbow. These two causes can be easily distinguished. In a true tennis elbow, the extension of the wrist joint is painful. During this test the elbow must be fully stretched. In a true tennis elbow, the side bending of the wrist towards the thumb side is also painful. Sometimes muscles on the lateral aspect of the forearm feel tender on deep palpation; these muscles help in extension at the wrist joint.

Treatment

A tennis elbow recovers on its own without any treatment in

about a year, if a person is under sixty years. However it takes longer when the person is over sixty.

Ordinarily it is treated by local hydrocortisone injections. These injections inhibit spontaneous recovery. It is not uncommon for patients to remain well after an injection for a few months and then feel the need for further injections month after month. If left untreated however, there is a possibility that the patient may recover completely in twelve months on his own.

Manipulation

Manipulation is found to be effective for a tennis elbow. The elbow is fixed and deep friction is applied on the epicondyl for five to ten minutes before manipulation. This softens the scar tissue which becomes easier to break by manipulation. Manipulation is repeated once or twice a week for four to six weeks. Such sessions are enough to relieve the pain completely. Manipulation is done in hyperextension. One may hear the cracking sound during manipulation and relief is felt immediately following the manipulation.

Manipulation shortens the time required for recovery, and once the condition is cured, it does not recur.

Case Histories

❑ A fifty-two-year old man with a good build, employed as a supervisor in building construction, had pain in the elbow for two months. He used to drive a motor cycle for an average of 100 km daily. But the pain made him incapable of driving., He even had a lot of difficulty in lifting and moving the telephone. He had stiffness in the elbow in the mornings, and was not able to sleep well due to the pain. He had had a similar pain earlier on and it had subsided with local injection of hydrocortisone.

X-rays and laboratory tests were conducted after the problem was diagnosed as a tennis elbow. He felt relief after the first manipulative treatment. The pain decreased gradually and subsided six weeks later. He was advised to use his arm as little

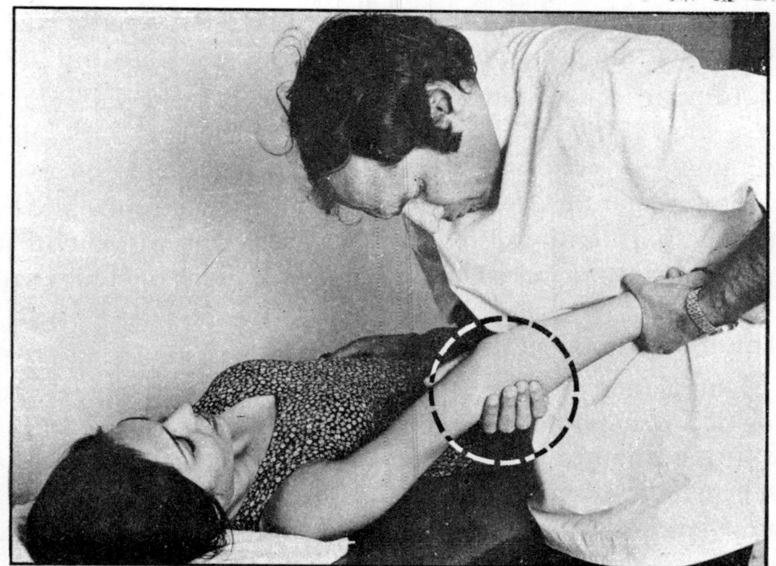

Fig. 41. A tennis elbow. *Overextending the patient's elbow as part of treatment.*

as possible during the treatment. He never complained of pain for two years following the treatment.

❑ A forty-one-year old housewife with five children had pain in the right elbow for five years. The pain had begun following a fall where she had supported herself by the hand. There was a slight swelling over the elbow. She experienced more pain if she used her hand more during work. Sometimes she felt pain in the forearm and upper arm upto the shoulder and neck.

She came to me with the above-mentioned complaint. There was a slight swelling over her left elbow. The X-ray showed no abnormality and the laboratory tests were normal.

Manipulation of the left elbow was started, along with manipulation of the cervical spine. She felt better following the first treatment. By the third week she was comfortable. The pain became more localised, and there was no pain in the neck and shoulder. The pain in the elbow subsided gradually and in ten weeks she was free of it.

11
Curing Wrist and Hand Pain

In most cases of pain in the wrist and hand, cervical manipulation is the treatment of choice. Patients respond rapidly to the treatment and all symptoms disappear within two or three weeks.

Pain in the wrist and hand may be due to varied factors. These may be:

- A mechanical disturbance in the cervical spine.
- Pressure on the median nerve as it passes in front of the wrist between the tunnel formed by the small bones of the wrist called carpal bones.
- Arthritis of the wrist joint.
- Post-traumatic or following the union of fractured bones of the wrist and hand.
- Often pain along with a tingling sensation and numbness in the fingers may radiate from the cervical spine. When the thumb is painful, the sixth cervical nerve may be involved. When the middle and index fingers are painful, this may be due to the involvement of the seventh cervical nerve. When the little finger is painful, this may be due to the eighth cervical nerve.

Carpal Tunnel Syndrome

The median nerve passes anteriorly in the wrist through the tunnel formed by the small bones of the wrist. It provides nerve supply to three and a half fingers of the hand (the thumb, index finger, middle finger and half of the ring finger). When this nerve is compressed while passing through the tunnel — numbness, a tingling sensation, and pain are caused in these fingers. This condition is most common in women of middle age. In the early stages, it occurs for short periods but may become continuous later. It is more severe at night and patients may wake up due to a distressing tingling in the hand, and may have to work the fingers and shake the hand to get relief. There is clumsiness in carrying out finger movements. Sewing and stitching become difficult. If the condition persists for a long time, weakness and a wasting of the small muscles of the hand which are supplied by the median nerve occurs.

A young woman had an acute pain in the neck, which subsided in course of time, but tingling, numbness and pain persisted in the thumb. Anti-inflammatory drugs decreased the pain and other symptoms. Fifteen days later she returned with the same numbness, tingling and pain in the first three and a half fingers. She also complained of pain over the wrist on exertion of pressure. She was injected with cortisone in the carpal tunnel, and felt a lot better for three weeks. Then the pain reappeared.

She came to me with the above history. I manipulated her cervical spine, articulated and mobilised her wrist and hand, and strapped her wrist to provide partial immobilisation. She felt considerable relief. This treatment was repeated once more after one week and she was completely cured after the third treatment, never again complaining of the same problem.

In my practice, I have treated quite a few cases of pain that has persisted for 5-10 years with apparent wasting of the small muscles of the hand. In such cases treatment was continued for 2-3 months. The results were encouraging: there was a persistent improvement in pain and decrease in muscle wasting. Arthritis and post-fracture pain in the wrist, and numbness in the fingers responded well to articulatory and manipulative treatment of the hand, followed by strapping.

Diagnosis

To differentiate between a cervical disc lesion and pressure on the median nerve in the carpal tunnel is sometimes difficult. The history of the course of the disease is informative.

Carpal tunnel pain increases with the use of the hand. The pain is located at the anterior aspect of the first three and a half fingers; there is no numbness above the wrist, though it might ache.

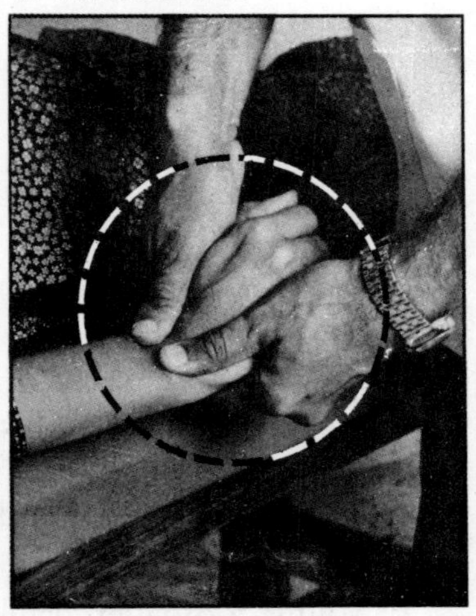

Fig. 42. Manipulation of the wrist joint.

In a cervical disc lesion, the patient feels pins and needles come and go day or night in an erratic manner, lasting not more than half an hour to one hour at a time. If the arm is elevated and held in that position for 2-3 minutes, numbness and tingling occur in 20-30 seconds.

In a few cases where diagnosis is not easy, improvement following manipulation helps to make a correct diagnosis.

Wasting and weakness of the hand muscles do not usually occur in cases which are detected early. In quite a few cases where surgery is performed, the cause of the compression on the nerve is not always known, the nerve and other structures appearing to be normal.

Treatment

Articulation of the wrist and hand followed by strapping gives encouraging results. In case of a cervical involvement, the cervical spine should be manipulated.

Contraindication. Manipulation of the hand and wrist are not done in cases of rheumatoid arthritis.

12
Relieving Knee Pain

Young or old, athletes or sedentary workers — most people get knee pain at some time or other. An old lady went crying to the doctor: 'I cannot walk; even walking in the house hurts me. I do not want to be crippled and dependent for little things on my children.' Old age and knee pain are almost synonymous.

A young footballer trying to kick the ball, fell down, but rose up and collecting all his courage, continued with the game. The next day, he had a big swelling over the knee and a lot of pain. He hobbled to the clinic with the help of a friend, was treated and asked to spend a few days in bed. For several weeks he limped in great discomfort. The pain and swelling gradually subsided. A few months later he complained of pain in the knee whenever he exerted it. It would swell up for a day or two after the strain and the swelling would subside completely a few days later. If the legs were stretched to their full, they hurt, and sometimes he found it difficult to bend the knee joints. Rotational movements at the knee also hurt. All this indicated that the ligaments had been strained during the injury and adhesions had formed during recovery. Due to the pain, the knee was not being used to its full extent, and following this, wasting of the thigh muscles had started, further aggravating the pain.

Weak muscles are not able to give full support to the knee and all the strain falls upon the ligaments. What is the treatment for such a knee? The answer lies in breaking the adhesions by manipulative reduction: this will bring back free and painless movement. The patient should be advised to do exercises for the quadriceps and rebuild his thigh muscles to give the knee full support. Strong thigh muscles take off the strain from the ligaments and the pain disappears completely. If the ligaments undergo a long stress and are stretched for long, they start aching. Muscles can remain contracted for any length of time and they will not ache.

The knee is the largest joint in the body, and has the function of supporting the entire body weight. One of the disadvantages of the knee joint is that it does not heal quickly. For faster healing any joint should be given proper rest. This is not possible for the knee joint. As you get up, stand and walk, you put all the weight of the body on your knees and irritate the healing joint.

However the knee is a joint where a more exact diagnosis can be made than in any other joint because the greater part of the joint and its ligaments and tendons can be felt by the hands.

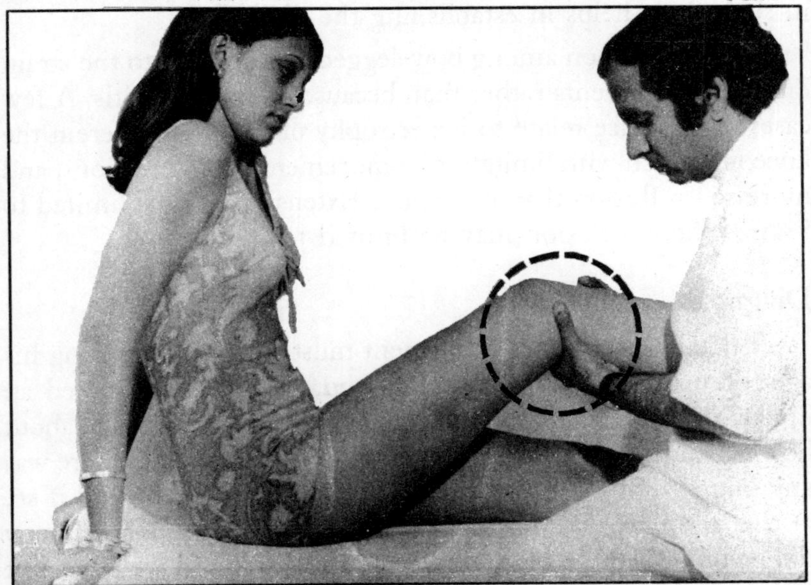

Fig. 43. Manipulation for pain in the knee.

Sometimes when diagnosis is not possible in a middle-aged person, the cause of pain may be a cartilagenous loose body inside the joint. Cartilage cannot be seen in an X-ray picture. Sometimes bone margins can flake off as loose bodies and be seen in the X-ray, but most of the time they are not the cause of pain as they remain attached to the synovial membrane of the joint capsule and do not cause any interference in movement.

The pain is often localised in the joint itself. An impacted loose body in the joint may cause pain, thus complicating an existent case of osteoarthritis. The pain may be up in the thigh and down in the leg but the patient quite clearly indicates that the symptoms originate from the knee.

Pain in front of the knee can also be caused by a lesion in the lower back. Any mechanical disturbance at the third lumbar nerve may cause pain in the knee. In such cases a patient complains of vague pain in the whole knee and cannot pin-point the exact spot. He may complain of pain above the knee cap or in front, or in the inner aspect of the thigh upto the groin. The hip joint, when at fault, can also cause pain in the knee. Examination of the knee in such cases helps in establishing the diagnosis.

Pain is common among bow-legged persons due to the strain on certain ligaments rather than because of osteoarthritis. A few cases of the knee relate to hypertrophy of the joint wherein the knee is swollen with limitation of movement in all directions, and more so on flexion than extension. Extension may be limited to 5-10°, whereas flexion may be limited to 60-90°.

Diagnosis

A detailed history of the patient must be taken including his age, occupation, how the pain started, whether he suffered an injury, and if so, in what position. Enquiries must be made about how he was standing, how he twisted his knee, whether there was any injury at all. Did the knee give way? Did it lock, and if so, at that time, was the leg straight or bent? If it was locked, how did he unlock it? Was the pain located all over? Did the pain shift from one place to another? Did the knee swell, and if so, how

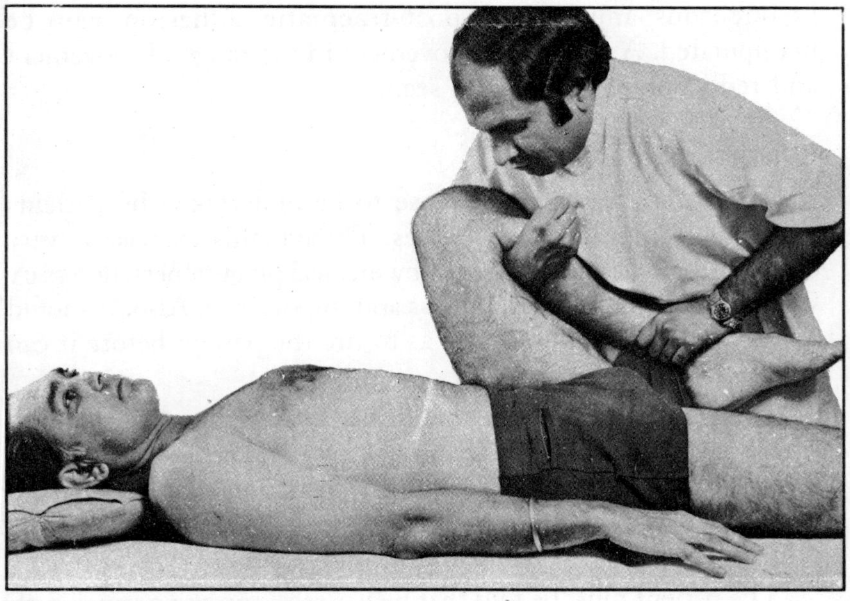

Fig. 44. Manipulation of the knee joint.

quickly? For how long was the patient disabled? Was he still experiencing sudden twinges, feeling clicks or hearing grating sounds in the knee?

The diagnosis has to be clear before treatment is started, the X-rays and laboratory tests confirming the diagnosis. However, the following conditions must also be excluded before manipulating a joint: a tubercular knee, gonorrheal or septic arthritis, gout, rheumatoid arthritis, active infective arthritis and other possible ailments.

Treatment

Manipulative reduction helps in complete recovery in the shortest period. Manipulation helps to achieve full movement at the knee joint. Realignment of the joint bones takes off all the strain from the ligaments, and they recover completely. Manipulation can be done on the young and the old. Techniques and manoeuvres are selected according to the needs of the patient. All cases of advanced osteoarthritis, chronic ligamentous injury and post-traumatic adhesion can be manipulated. A gradual improvement in the range of movement and reduction in the pain is seen.

Quadriceps Drill

This is an important exercise to be undertaken by patients suffering from pain in the knees. Though this exercise is very commonly advocated to patients by medical practitioners, necessary stress is not laid on its usefulness and importance. Also, it should not be done so strenuously so as to tire the patient before it can be effective.

The girth of the thigh should be measured and the patient should be educated about the *wasting* and *weakness* of his muscles. This can be measured by making a mark three or four inches above the upper margin of the knee cap and girth of both the thighs measured and compared in both legs.

The patient must be told that he has to regain the normal girth and strength and that this will take time. It cannot be achieved in a week or a month; it will take a couple of months or even a year. At each visit the girth of the thigh must be measured and noted so as to make the patient more conscious of this.

The quadriceps drill must be done in the following manner:

The patient is asked to lie on his back keeping his leg straight. He is asked to contract and tighten the thigh muscles without bending the knee. As he contracts his thigh muscles, the knee cap is seen moving up and down. This has to be done for 2-3 minutes at a time and repeated during the day as often as possible, preferably 20 times a day. This simple exercise can be done while standing or sitting. To do this while sitting, one has to place oneself on the edge of the chair, straighten the leg and keep the back of the heel on the ground. It can then be done comfortably. The patient gets into the habit of doing this exercise without any effort in seven to ten days' time. It becomes as effortless as cycling or driving. It is so convenient that it can be done in the office, at home, or even while waiting for the bus.

This exercise starts showing results in three to four weeks.

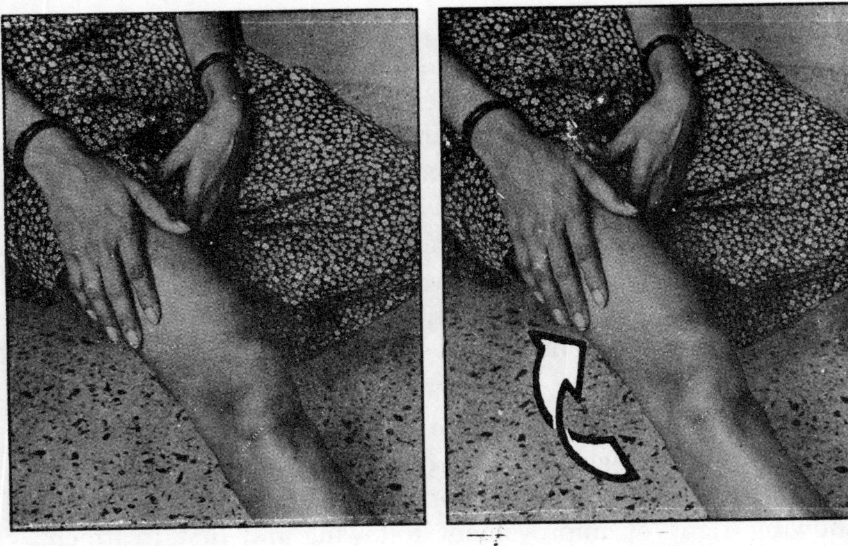

Fig. 45. Quadriceps drill. *A. Relaxed position;* B. *Thigh muscles contracted; the knee cap is automatically raised.*

Weight Reduction

All the body weight has to be carried by the knee joint. A reduction in weight relieves it of the pressure to some extent.

The medical practitioner asks the patients to walk as much as they can and keep their joints mobile, so that they do not get jammed. In my opinion, movement is desirable, but not the strain of walking when the pain is severe. As the pain decreases, the patient can undertake further activity.

The strain of standing can be taken off from the knee if the patient is asked to bend the painful knee and put it on a chair or stool and stand on the painless leg, for instance, while washing at the basin or cleaning utensils. This will protect the painful knee from excessive strain and give it rest so as to hasten the recovery period.

Case Histories

- A forty-year-old man in the tea business was involved in a car accident and had pain in his left knee. It subsided after taking shortwave diathermy and doing knee exercises for about a month. However the pain in the knee continued to come and go, and gradually increased. For one and a half months it became almost continuous. It was painful for the patient to get up after sitting on the ground. The pain became worse and reached the thigh. Due to this and lack of activity, he began gaining weight and added six kilograms to his weight. The X-ray of the damaged knee showed osteoarthritis.

Manipulative treatment of the left knee was started. The knee was strapped following manipulation. The patient was asked to do the quadriceps drill for forty minutes a day. He began showing signs of improvement following the first treatment and the pain became much less by the end of the third week. He recovered in two months, and was advised to continue the exercise for another month.

- A 65-year-old lady had pain in the left knee for three years. Later on the pain started in the right knee too, and was accompanied by pain in the lower back with numbness and tingling. She consulted an orthopaedic surgeon and five injections of hydrocortisone were given inside the knee joint. These helped her and she felt better. After two months however, the pain started all over again and she went to her village and underwent massage for two and a half months. She did get relief but the pain persisted.

When she came to me, the X-rays of her lumbar spine and both knees indicated that she suffered from osteoarthritis. The lumbo-sacral spine showed a slipped disc with osteoarthritic changes.

After manipulative treatment for the lumbar spine and both knee joints, she was advised to do the quadriceps exercise at home every day. She started showing improvement from the second week. The pain in her lower back and the tingling sensation in the left leg subsided in six weeks and her knees showed considerable improvement. She made complete recovery in three months.

- A fifty-seven-year-old lady, obese but tall, had a job which compelled her to walk long distances. She began experiencing pain in the left knee though she had not suffered any injury. She felt more pain and stiffness when she tried to get up after sitting for a while. The pain became severe for ten days. She took anti-inflammatory drugs but these did not help. Local application of ointments and heat from an infrared lamp did not help either.

The X-ray showed osteoarthritis. Manipulative treatment of the left knee was done followed by strapping and the quadriceps exercise. She started feeling better after the third visit. By the end of seven weeks she got rid of her symptoms.

13

Curing Leg, Ankle and Foot Pain

I was working as the Registrar in the Emergency Department of the Southend-on-Sea General Hospital in England, when one morning, I received a phone call from a local practitioner. He told me that his wife had slipped and sprained her ankle while descending the steps at home, and he wanted me to examine her. She came to my department with a limp. She was not able to put complete pressure on her affected foot. It was swollen and it appeared that she was in terrible pain. I examined her and then asked for an X-ray. The X-ray revealed no fracture in the foot and by looking at it, it appeared that nothing was abnormal. This was a simple case of a sprained ankle. When her husband arrived, I told him my findings and suggested that if I could manipulate her ankle joint, recovery would be fast. He agreed and I administered manipulative treatment to her foot. Following the manipulation, I strapped the foot for support and asked her to report back after three days. I was surprised when she walked in after three days without a limp. She had already taken off the strappings. The swelling had disappeared and she had no pain at all. Her happiness clearly indicated that she had never expected her foot to recover so fast. A recovery which could have taken three weeks and might have lasted as chronic pain and inconvenience for months or years, was completely cured.

The foot is an example of mechanical perfection. It bears the whole body weight and is often the site of pain, next in frequency only to backache. The following movements occur at the ankle joint:

Upward movement of the foot called dorsiflexion

Downward movement of the foot called planter flexion

Inward movement of the foot called inversion

Outward movement of the foot called eversion

The ankle joint is classified as a hinge joint. The talus or ankle-bone wedged between the lateral malleolus (fibula) and medial malleolus (tibia) receives superimposed weight from the tibia. Dorsiflexion and planter flexion are major movements at the ankle joint. Eversion and inversion are negligible. Inversion and eversion movements are carried out mainly at foot joints or tarsal joints. These movements are better visualised by putting the foot firmly on the floor for bearing weight.

The arrangement of bones in the foot is such that it constitutes different arches in the foot. They are the medial arch, the lateral arch, and the transverse arches.

The medial arch can be seen on the inner aspect of the foot while standing. It gives the foot a springing action and makes the foot more flexible and supple. The arches of the foot bear the weight of the whole body.

Common causes of pain at the ankle joint and the foot are sprains, flat feet, bursitis of the sole, calcaneal spur and bad shoes.

Sprained Ankle

A sprained ankle is one of the most common problems. It involves multiple joints in the foot and more than one ligament gets sprained. In due course one joint may recover, leaving chronic disability in another. This is the reason why many a time a sprained ankle does not heal completely and pain persists, which is not acute but enough to bother the individual and make a long walk uncomfortable.

In most cases the ankle gets sprained due to a sudden inward movement of the whole foot. All the bones of the foot do not return to their normal position after a sprain. Instead there is

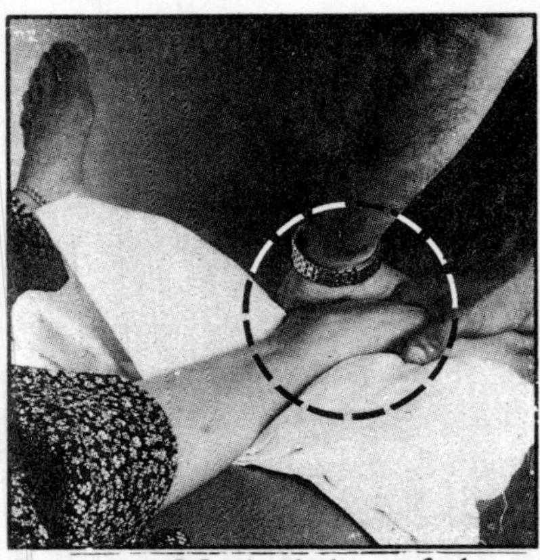
Fig. 46. Manipulation of the ankle joint and foot.

tautness in a particular ligament which does not heal and sometimes gets lengthened, causing chronic pain and making the ankle joint hypermobile in a particular direction. Manipulation of a sprained ankle helps the alignment of the foot bones and releases all the tension from the ligament. Recovery is spontaneous and complete. But many patients do not get this treatment and in its absence, suffer from a disability, a constant discomfort and nagging pain which reduces the ability of the foot to support the body, thereby reducing its suppleness. Sometimes deep massage done with the tip of the index finger or thumb on the aching ligament, for 10-15 minutes, 3-4 times a week, helps in complete recovery.

Treatment. If the pain is acute and the ankle joint has considerable swelling, manipulation is not done for 2-3 days till the swelling has subsided substantially. When the swelling is slight, manipulation can be done. After manipulation, strapping is done to give the foot necessary support.

When the foot is sprained due to a sudden inward movement, after articulating and relaxing the muscles of the ankle joint, strapping is done in such a way as to maintain the foot in slight eversion.

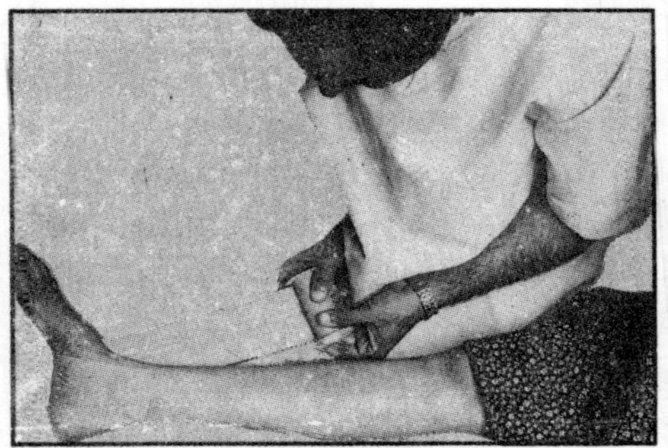
Fig. 47. Strapping the ankle joint.

Keeping the foot in a bucketful of warm saline water, and moving the foot and ankle joint under water in all possible directions, helps to reduce the swelling faster and regain mobility. Trying to walk on the inner edge of foot is sometimes very helpful.

Chronic Case. An injured foot may face no problem while used for ordinary purposes, but may swell up and ache after vigorous and prolonged use. This means that a scar has been allowed to form in the process of incomplete healing. Treatment consists of manipulative rupture of the scar adhesions. This is a simple process and does not need any anaesthesia. One sharp twist articulating the foot, often accompanied by a crack, is enough to cure a patient completely in most cases.

Flat Foot

This is a fairly common condition. The longitudinal arch of the foot is reduced. When a patient stands, the inner border of the foot is in contact with the ground. A flat foot is usually associated with a slight outward twisting of the foot. Sometimes it is hereditary or due to muscle weakness; at other times, there is no apparent cause.

All children have flat feet at the age of one to two years when they start to stand. Sometimes this deformity persists in adult life. Many children with flat feet do not complain of any pain but the shoes persistently bulge inwards and the heels wear off more quickly on the inner side. Some adults may have no symptom. A few experience an ache after walking. Manipulation helps a lot in a painful flat foot, but often has to be repeated every week for a couple of months. Alteration in shoes also helps in such cases.

The shoe should be tilted slightly on the outer side by inserting a wedge base medially in-between the layer of the heel (not the sole). This helps the inner twist and reduces the bulging of the shoes.

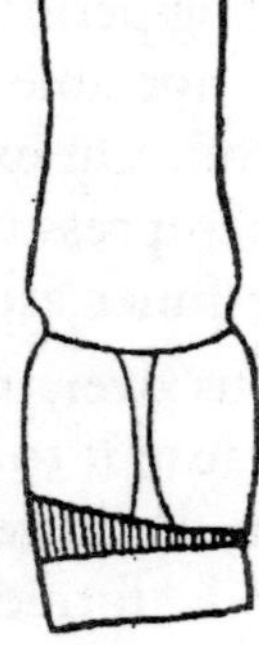

Fig. 48. Inner wedge added to the heel of a shoe in case of a flat foot.

In older children and adults, a few exercises are advised to strengthen the foot muscles. They are as follows:

1. Walking on the outer border of the foot.

2. Trying to lift glass balls from the ground with the help of the toes and the forefoot.

3. Spreading out a small towel on the ground and trying to pull it near the foot with the help of the forefoot and toes.

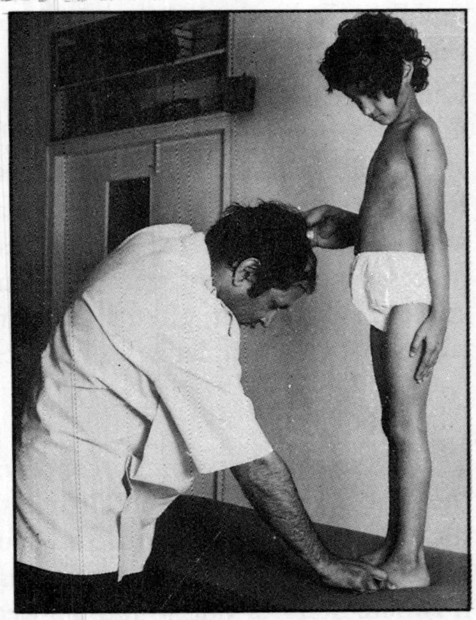

Fig. 49. Assessing the severity of flat feet.

Fascitis and Calcaneal Spur

Many patients complain of pain in the sole or the heel when walking and standing; they do not feel any pain while sitting and lying down. The pain is more severe when the patient gets up in the morning and puts his feet on the ground. He feels a little better after moving around for a while. While standing, the shape of the foot is maintained partly by the muscles. When the patient stands for a long period, however, this tires the muscles of the feet and they are not able to carry the burden of weight and soon become painful. On examination, the feet appear to be normal. But when deep pressure is applied by the fingers, they may feel tender at the inner aspect of the sole and the heel.

Continuous overstrain on the fascia (a thin sheet of fibrous tissue) may cause it to be pulled away from its origin at the heel or calcaneum. Periosteum being the outermost covering of the bone, a gap is formed which gets filled up with new bone formation often termed as a calcanean spur.

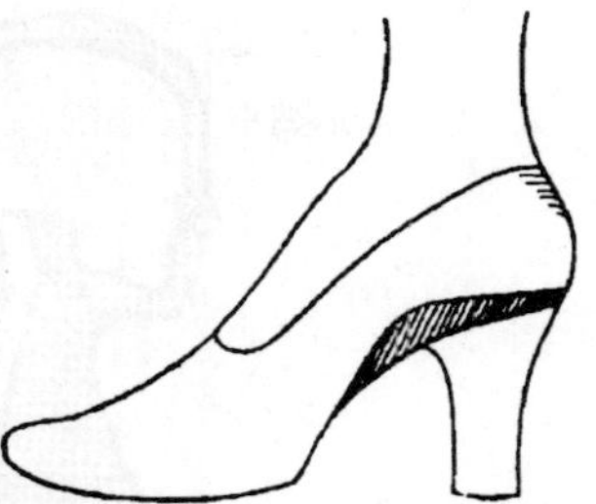

Fig. 50. *Shoemakers offer different heights of heel catering to the osteopath's instructions. Heels are kept horizontal.*

A calcanean spur may occur without any pain in some patients, while many patients complain of pain without any spur formation. Once the spur is formed, it is permanent and even after the pain is completely cured, the spur remains.

Treatment

Manipulation of feet is helpful. This may have to be repeated a number of times at weekly intervals depending upon the severity of the pain.

Wearing a specially designed shoe where the heel and forefoot are brought nearer, thus relaxing the fascia of the sole, may provide relief. The heel is raised keeping its upper surface horizontal. The height of the heel is determined by asking the patient to stand on a wooden platform with varying levels of thickness, until the minimum height of the heel that removes the symptom is found. A correct-sized heel provides immediate relief. Now the short flexor muscles of the sole are energetically treated with exercise and deep friction. Manipulation is of the greatest advantage as it secures mobility in different joints of the foot.

Selecting Shoes

Footwear can be a cause of pain in the feet. Shoes must be selected considering the weight distribution and mechanism of the feet. Badly designed shoes not only hurt for a while, but become a cause of constant pain. Ladies' shoes with high heels and pointed toes are particularly to be blamed.

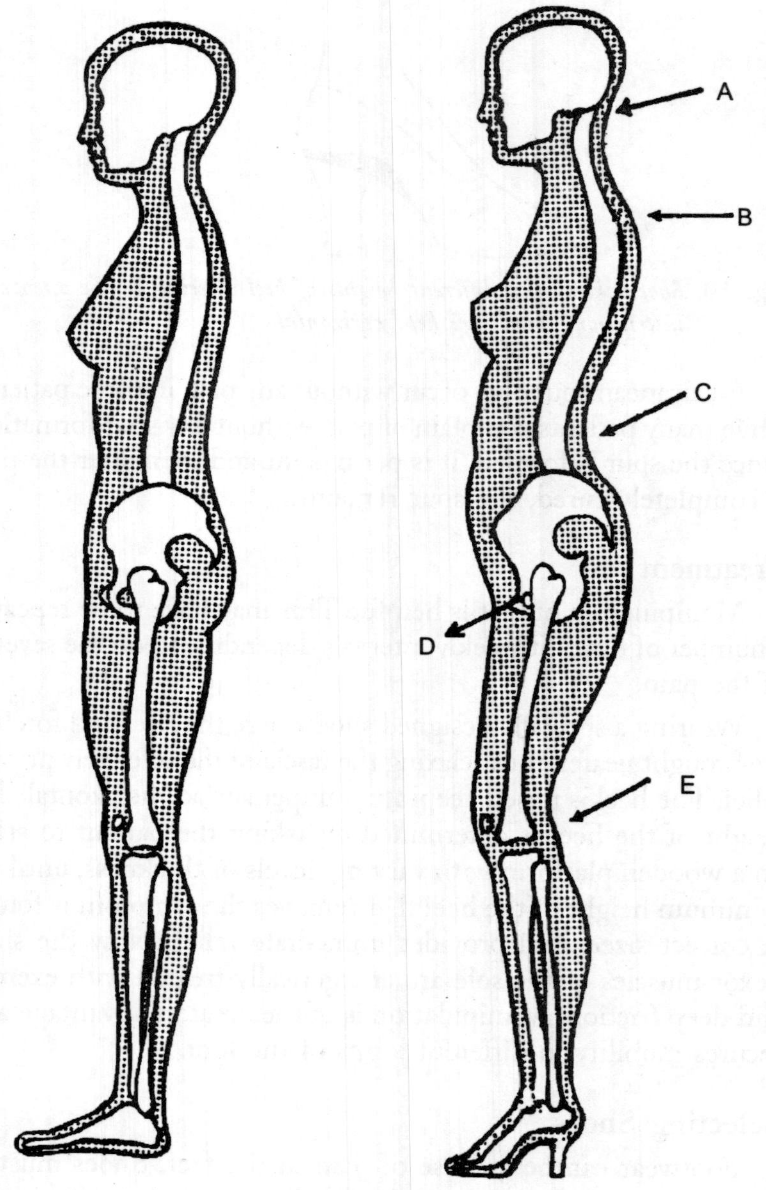

Fig. 51. Footwear may cause pain in the A. *Neck;* B. *Upper back;* C. *Lower back;* D. *Hip;* E. *Knee or foot. High heels are not healthy. Choose your shoes carefully.*

Case History

- ❑ A 39-year-old man, doing business in tyres, jumped from a height of six feet while drunk. He fractured three bones in his right ankle and had to use a plaster for three months following manipulation under general anaesthesia. After the removal of the plaster, an X-ray was taken once again; it showed a complete union of the bones. But the pain persisted after the removal of the plaster. Even a little walking would cause swelling and pain. The patient consulted a few orthopaedic surgeons. One of them advised an operation and fusion of the bones; others were against such an operation.

The patient was not able to sleep and began taking pain relieving and sleeping pills. He was frustrated because he was unable to look after his business properly.

He then came to me. After articulation and manipulation of the ankle, strappings were applied to give support to the joint. In three months he was ninety-five per cent fit and could walk without getting any swelling or pain. He went about his business and daily routine without much difficulty.

14
Relieving Old Age Problems

A few old-age symptoms respond well to manipulative therapy. Persons of fifty years of age and over experience some stiffness of the cervical spine. They feel disturbed while sleeping, putting the blame on the faulty position of their sleeping pillow or prolonged fatigue. Sometimes a little disturbance is sufficient to bring about a headache. It may be caused by bad posture or a wrong way of doing work or inactivity. Relief is felt by taking a painkiller or by applying warm water to the upper back. Such people find difficulty in balancing themselves, and are afraid of crossing the road on their own. They feel as if they are going to fall down. They feel giddy when they turn their head to one side or while bending it backwards. They may have ringing in the ear, or suffer a hearing loss. They feel as if they have specks of dust in front of their eyes. Occasionally they may also experience difficulty in speaking or hoarseness, hot flushes or perspiration. Nose or eye secretions may increase or decrease.

Psychic disturbances among old people are very common. They complain of mental fatigue, difficulty in concentration, loss of memory, depression and anxiety. These symptoms can occur in various combinations and with a varying degree of intensity.

Results of Manipulation

Giddiness and headache respond very well to manipulation. Fatigue in the eyes improves to a considerable degree. Manipulation has a good effect on nose and eye secretions too. Ear noises can be lessened a little bit, but the results are not satisfactory. Sometimes these patients are forced to take psychiatric treatment. Dr Feld, a neurosurgeon, drew attention to disturbances of cervical origin. These symptoms are now accepted as being related to vertebral artery insufficiency; cervical manipulation is justified in these cases.

Case History

❑ A 74-year-old lady suffered from stiffness and occasional pain in the neck. Both shoulders used to pain and this went on for several years. She had spells of giddiness lasting for a few minutes each. On a few occasions she was semi-conscious for about ten minutes to half an hour. She did not remember things and her sleep was disturbed.

The patient was treated with articulation and mild manipulation of the cervical spine. Her giddiness became less frequent, and she became more alert. She could move around in the house more easily and did not need help. She also felt relief from her shoulder pain.

15
Diet, Hydrotherapy and Yoga

Why do we ask gout patients to abstain from meat and alcoholic drinks? Why do we experience relief in knee pain when our bowels move well? Why is smoking prohibited in cases of intermittent claudication (cramping pain in the leg caused by arterial obstruction) and coronary heart disease?

There is no controversy about the fact that the body has its own resistance, and it fights against all diseases. Why then do we not adopt methods and means to increase the body's own resistance?

There is much abuse of drugs. Patients suffering from pain for years are put on strong, stronger and the strongest drugs till they fall victim to them. They experience many side-effects such as a peptic ulcer, gastritis, and deteriorated liver and kidney function.

Food has a great role to play in causing and alleviating pain in different diseases. The father of modern medicine, Hippocrates, said: 'Let medicine be thy food, and food, thy medicine.' Proper food helps in stopping the abuse of drugs.

The use of water, the sun, natural food, a correct diet, physical exercise and yoga is a help in providing relief in various diseases. Osteopathy believes in treating the body as a whole.

A vegetarian diet, as well as the inclusion of fruits, green vegetables and salad in our food are vital. Fried food and spices should be avoided as far as possible. Physical exercise keeps us healthy. Drinking a lot of water helps to flush the kidneys. Fruits, vegetables and salad in our diet provide vitamins and minerals and help in bowel movement.

Water is used in its three forms: ice, water and steam. We apply ice to bleeding vessels; they constrict and the bleeding stops. When a steam bath is given to a patient with a backache, it relaxes his muscles and offers pain relief. This is what we call hydrotherapy.

Tension does have an effect on headaches and cervical spondylosis. Tension and worries tighten the muscles of the neck and the upper back and shoulders, and this aggravates the pain by increasing the lesion at the level of the cervical spine. Therefore meditation is of prime importance to learn to relax the mind and body.

Yoga has been used for millennia in India. It is an excellent antidote against the ills brought about by too much stress. Excessive stress can cause many psysiological problems. Yoga has proved its efficacy in tackling such problems, and is becoming increasingly popular even in the west.

A system of self-treatment, the malfunctioning of the body system due to bad habits, incorrect food intake, and a faulty lifestyle can be cured with *yoga.*

If *yoga asanas* are done as a routine throughout life, the muscles will not grow. Digestion will improve, sleep will be sound, sight will become sharp, and hearing will become more sensitive. This will happen because *asanas* assist the nervous system and endocrine glands to improve their functioning.

To sum up, a healthy daily routine and a proper diet protect one from disease and promote good health.

Glossary

Ankylosing spondylitis. Inflammation of the spine, limiting movement.

Antisepsis. The process of preventing bacteria from growing.

Bamboo spine. A spine lacking in mobility; it looks like a knotted bamboo in an X-ray.

Brachial neuralgia. Inflammation of the nerves at the shoulder.

Chiropractic. The diagnosis and manipulative treatment of mechanical disorders of the joints, especially of the spinal column.

Cholecystitis. Inflammation of the gall bladder.

Collagenous. Made of collagen, a cementing substance consisting of protein, and present between the cells.

Condyl. The lower end of the thigh bone.

Coronary thrombosis. A blockage of the blood flow caused by a blood clot in a coronary artery.

Enuresis. Loss of control over passing urine.

Epicondyl. Cartilagenous covering over the condyl.

Fascia. A thin sheet of tissue.

Fibrositis. Inflammation of the fibrous tissue.

Foramen. An opening, especially in a bone.

Histamine. A substance secreted in the body, which dilates the blood vessels and is produced more in an allergic reaction.

Hyaline. A thin whitish sheet of tissue.

Hydrostatic pressure. Pressure exerted by water or a fluid on the walls of the containing vessel.

Hypertrophy. The enlargement of an organ or tissue due to an increase in its body cells.

Kyphosis. An excessive outward curvature of the spine, causing hunching of the back.

Lordosis. An inward curvature of the spine, giving the appearance of bending backwards.

Mucosaccarides. A lubricating substance in the bony joints.

Myocardial infarction. Necrosis or death of the heart muscle due to stoppage of blood supply to it.

Myositis. Inflammation of muscle tissue.

Occipital. The back part of the skull.

Osteomyelitis. Inflammation of the bone.

Osteophytes. Excess bone formation inside a joint.

Periarthritis. Inflammation around the joint.

Prophylaxis. Preventive measures.

Sacro-iliac. Pertaining to the sacrum, the last part of the spine, and ileum, the upper part of the hip bone.

Sclerosis. Scar formation.

Synovial fluid. A lubricating fluid secreted inside a bony joint space.

Hot Water Therapy

Dr. Patrick Horay & David Harp

If you ever suffer from:

- Tension headaches from stress
- Chronic backache from hours of desk-work
- Sprains and strains from weekend sports
- Injuries from accidents
- Painful joints and muscles due to over-exertion aging or inactivity

Hot Water Therapy can help.

This book will introduce you to simple, effective techniques you can use while relaxing in your shower, bath, or hot tub to relieve pain and strengthen aching muscles. And they take only a few minutes to do!

You will learn that you can save your "bad back" by using a combination of gentle massage, exercise and stretching. When you blend these routines with the soothing, healing qualities of hot water, you'll enjoy the age-old benefits of spa treatment — right in your own bathroom.

Illustrated pp 152

Nature Cure for Common Diseases

Vithaldas Modi

"Comprehensive ... presents in a simple straight forward and convincing manner the advantages of Nature Cure or Naturopathy in aiding recovery from all acute and chronic ailments and conditions and in maintaining health and vitality."

Hindustan Times

"... contains many useful hints for the layman, both for the prevention and cure of ailments."

Bhavan's Journal

"The most welcome aspect of naturopathy is that it does away with pills and nostrums."

Indian Express

PP 200

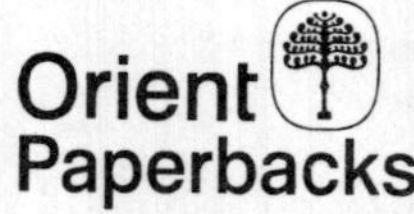

5A/8, Ansari Road, New Delhi-110 002
www.orientpaperbacks.com